Promoting Community Mental Health

Paula Worby
Todd Jailer

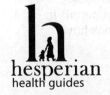

hesperian
health guides

Oakland, California USA

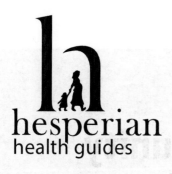

hesperian
health guides

Published by:
Hesperian Health Guides
2860 Telegraph Avenue
Oakland, California 94609 USA
www.hesperian.org

Copyright © 2025 by Hesperian Health Guides
Second printing: August 2025
First English edition: February 2025
ISBN: 978-0-942364-02-6
First ebook edition: February 2025
ISBN: 978-0-942364-13-2

Help us improve this book!

We developed this book by learning from people implementing creative community-based mental health approaches. Your feedback will help make future editions better.

Contact us at: MentalHealth@hesperian.org to tell us how you are using this book and what you think.

This book was printed in the USA by EPAC.

Credits

Editorial oversight: Sarah Shannon
Additional writing: Maria Seymour St. John, Linda Spangler, Sarah Shannon
Additional editing: Amy Hill, Cynthia Peters, Sarah Shannon
Project management and art coordination: Paula Worby
Design and production: Kathleen Tandy, Luis Aspeitia
Proofreading: Cynthia Peters
Index: Victoria Baker
Cover design: Kathleen Tandy, Rosemary Jason

Illustrations: We gratefully acknowledge the artists whose work illustrates this book: Akiko Aoyagi Shurtleff, Luis Aspeitia, Hana Barker, Sara Boore, Heidi Broner, Elizabeth Clark-Sutton, Regina Faul-Doyle, Sandy Frank, May Haddad, Jesse Hamm, Haris Ichwan, Rosemary Jason, Anna Kallis, Rodney Kawaayi, Susan McCallister, Lori Nadaskay, Gabriela Nuñez, Kimiye Owens, Nina Reimer, Petra Rohr-Rouendaal, Leana Rosetti, Chengyu Song, Kathleen Tandy, Dovile Tomkute-Veleckiene, Paul Tong, Lihua Wang, Christine Wong, Paula Worby, and Mary Ann Zapalac. Special thanks to Shu Ping Guan for her agile and skillful work.

Thanks

A debt of recognition to all current and former Hesperian staff and board involved in the development of our materials. Special thanks to: Jessica Barrera, Dani Behonick, Alicia Flores, Jade Fong, Samantha Heep, Zena Herman, Bill Lankford, Miriam Lara-Mejia, Meredith Larson, Aditi Malhotra, Susan McCallister, Kimiye Owens, Maile Robles, Melissa Smith, Keziah Sullivan, Dorothy Tegler, and Vanessa Tran. The 2025 reprint of this book was coordinated by Dani Behonick, with help from Luis Aspeitia, Amy Hill, Sarah Shannon, and Paula Worby.

We leaned heavily on a group of advisors who shared their wisdom and experience: M. Brinton Lykes, Maritza Martin, Sharoda McAllister, Baijayanta Mukhopadhyay, Maria Seymour St. John, Janey Skinner, Linda Spangler, Ariana Thompson-Lastad, and Aruna Uprety. This book would not have been possible without their early and ongoing support!

Our gratitude to the many people who generously shared insightful critiques, comments and guidance: Jessica Apfel, Dan Becker, Deborah Billings, America Bracho, S. Brooke Briggance, Mirna Cervantes, Natan Cohen, Galen Comerford, Sera Davidow, Keylin Figueroa, Juana Flores, Mariana Gonzalez, Andrea Heyward, Sally Hindman, Bill Joyce, Anna Kaminski, Jackie Leal, Ginger Lee, Reichi Lee, Christine Lewis, Hannah Mack, Marci Manderscheid, Jennifer Mineer, Ámate Perez, Mark Pohlman, Christian Radziwon, Brooke Riedlinger, Laura Rodriguez, Brenda Sanchez, Pamela Secada-Sales, Rajasee Sharma, Ruth Sherer, Vanessa Monique Smith, Julie Smithwick, Laura Snyder Brown, Esther Stauffer, Sophie Taggart, Laura Turiano, Kaethe Weingarten, and Sarah Zemore.

Special appreciation

Special appreciation to the community-based groups who contributed their hearts, time, and experiences to make this book as useful as possible:

Community Health Worker Institute (University of South Carolina Arnold School of Public Health), Domestic Workers United, Latino Health Access, Migrant Clinicians Network's Witness to Witness Program, Mujeres Unidas y Activas, Multicultural Institute, My Digital TAT2, Native American Health Center, Puente de la Costa Sur, Southeast Arizona Health Education Center (SEAHEC), Tiburcio Vasquez Health Center, Tiny Village Spirit, Wildflower Alliance, and The Women's Initiative.

Funders

Project funding from the Ittleson Foundation, West Foundation, Wyomissing Foundation and an anonymous donor was essential to bringing this resource to life. General support funding (covering a host of necessary activities and bridging gaps in project funding) was generously provided by the Cogan Family Foundation, Lakeshore Foundation, and individual donors to Hesperian Health Guides. We are deeply grateful for this support.

Acknowledgements

We thank and acknowledge the following sources:

The description of finger-holding (page 21) is adapted from the *CAPACITAR Emergency Response Tool Kit*, Patricia Mathes Cane (2005). While the concepts of "speak the unspeakable" and "protective shield," are part of child-parent psychotherapy, the related activities in this book (pages 36 and 39) were developed by Maria Seymour St. John, with inspiration from *Don't hit my mommy!: A manual for child-parent psychotherapy with young witnesses of family violence*, Lieberman, Alicia F., and Patricia Van Horn, Zero to Three (2005). "How to communicate with a person experiencing psychosis" (page 57) was developed by Maria Seymour St. John with information from Psychosis: First aid guidelines (mhfainternational.org/guidelines), Mental Health First Aid Australia (MHFA), Melbourne (2019) and *Implementing Early Intervention in Psychosis*, Edwards, J & McGorry, PD., Martin Dunitz, London (2002). "Chart your digital loop" (page 115) is adapted by Hesperian from materials kindly shared by My Digital TAT2. The activity "Find stress-busters" (page 151) is adapted from Chapter 12: Stress Management and Self Care by Joani Marinoff, from *Training Guide to Foundations for Community Health Workers*, Tim Berthold (ed.), Community Health Worker Certificate Program, City College of San Francisco (October 2015), and other useful ideas are provided in its accompanying textbook, *Foundations for Community Health Workers*.

Contents

Where to find

Introduction

Rarely, if ever, are any of us healed in isolation.
Healing is an act of communion. — bell hooks

Who is a mental health promoter? You are.

We all interact with people every day—in big and small ways—as friends, neighbors, workers, or volunteers. We listen, address shared problems, search for resources, and provide support. As we do this, we are already promoting community mental health.

We are often part of networks looking out for the community's safety, housing, food access, employment, interpersonal relationships, health care, and other aspects of health and well-being. This book was created to help strengthen community mental health through the work you are already doing.

If you are a social worker or peer counselor with training in handling individual mental health concerns, this book will encourage you to apply your experience to promote mental health at a community level.

If you are a community housing organizer, you have training or experience in dealing with a housing crisis, but maybe not so much with an emotional crisis. Without becoming a therapist, the ideas in this book can help prepare you for challenging emotional moments, equip you to get through them skillfully, and find ways to get support for yourself as you navigate stressful organizing work. Your efforts to improve your community also improve mental health through social change.

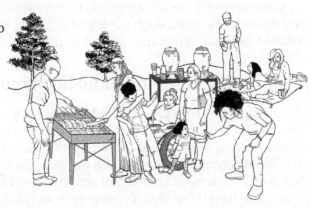

Recognizing and responding to emotional needs in a family, a group of friends, a neighborhood, or an organization is most often taken on by women. Women are asked to, expected to, and usually volunteer to step in and offer support. By encouraging and helping prepare everyone to respond to emotional needs and provide mental health support, we hope to lessen the emotional burden on women and improve their mental health too.

1

Mental health in our communities

Everything around us affects our mental health. Violence, discrimination, economic hardship, the climate crisis, widespread misinformation, and the feeling that things are getting worse instead of better—these affect what's on our mind, how we feel, and our health. At the same time, our lives and mental health are affected in positive ways by the kindness and supportive interactions of those around us. Feeling connected, having people we can talk with, being part of a community—these make us feel better about ourselves and our communities.

During times of crisis, people often become more aware of their own and others' mental health; for example, when people lose homes due to fires or floods, when a factory closing creates community unemployment, or when a school shooting creates fear among children and parents. This also happened during the COVID pandemic. People often respond to crisis by taking collective action to build up their communities—helping neighbors, creating mutual aid groups, and finding more ways to feel hope and purpose, and reduce isolation, anxiety, distress and loss.

Individual mental health

Everyone's life is filled with ups and downs, moments of both happiness and sadness. When you can handle daily life and its challenges, care for yourself and others, maintain your relationships, have a sense of purpose and feel like you "belong," your mental health is likely to be good. Mental health means feeling emotions but managing them, suffering from loss and disappointment but recovering, and adapting to changes.

When difficulties occur, they affect mental health by causing stronger than usual feelings of stress, worry, and sometimes even despair. That's when each person draws on their personal strengths and resilience. But we don't depend on ourselves alone: we also look to the ties of love and belonging we have built with family, friends, and supportive community.

Although every person responds to mental health stresses differently, and will find different paths through them and different kinds of support helpful, promoting community while promoting mental health benefits everyone.

It's all connected: Individual/community, physical/mental

US society views both physical and mental health issues as individual problems with individual solutions. Yet a person's physical and mental health respond to situations affecting groups and entire communities. While community organizing most often focuses on conditions determining physical health (like housing, food, safe streets, etc.), because physical and mental health are so interrelated, mental health improves at the same time. Likewise, a community mental health approach that targets social conditions will improve physical health.

ACTIVITY   **Making connections between individual and community mental health**

This group discussion of a city bus accident helps identify the connections among physical and mental health, individual and community health, and health and social conditions. Looking at all sides of a situation helps illuminate why community mental health promotion includes actions to benefit everyone, from the most affected to those affected in less visible ways.

1. Describe the event and its immediate effects: After a bus accident in a busy urban area, a few passengers might have broken bones, while others have only scrapes. Probably many more will have bruises that won't be visible until the next day, and may also feel sore for a few days. Everyone involved was frightened and some suffered a serious emotional shock. Other people in cars, on bicycles, or on the sidewalk might be affected too.

2. Lead a discussion reflecting on questions such as:

   Physical effects: What kinds of physical effects might passengers and others have from the crash? Which are visible and which are harder to see? How many people will get care for their injuries? How will it affect people's mental health to seek treatment for and possibly live with the long-term effects of their injuries?

   Mental health effects: What are different ways passengers and others might react to the frightening experience of the crash? Will some try to avoid thinking about it? Will others talk through the frightening experience with friends or family? Will some have nightmares about traffic accidents? How many people will get mental health care to help them process this event?

   What else might people experience? Will some refuse to take buses or bike in busy areas, and how will that affect their lives? Will people wonder if any changes will be made to prevent other accidents like this? And how will that affect the daily worries that people already manage?

ACTIVITY   Making connections between individual and community mental health *(continued)*

3. Ask the group to identify possible responses the transit company and local government might propose, and what responses the community would like to see:

Will the city transit company investigate the accident? Will they fire the driver who got into the accident? Will they improve driver training? Will the transit company better maintain the buses so they are safer to ride in? Will the local government make changes so the streets become less dangerous?

Will a community group engage in a transportation justice and accountability process? Will they look into whether: The oldest buses are used in poorer neighborhoods? If roads in poorer communities are less well-maintained? If there are fewer streetlights or traffic lights?

How would these actions—and the safer streets that could result—affect the physical and mental health of everyone in the community?

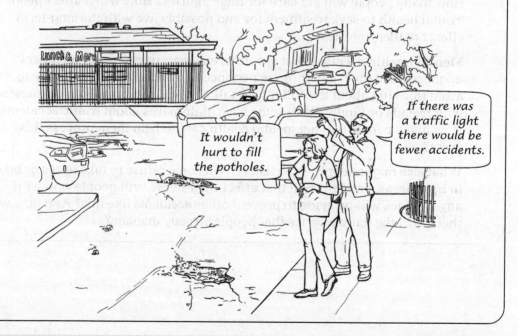

You can adapt this activity to discuss a different incident that happened (or could happen) in your community. Use similar questions that cover physical health, mental health, and economic and social conditions to explore how it would affect community mental health promotion.

How to use this book

You can find many self-help resources and books directed at professionals. But this book focuses on how community building and community organizing efforts can contribute to mental health. We feature groups that have taken action based on their specific community, its needs and strengths. We greatly appreciate them and their work, and encourage you to learn more about them from their websites (see pages 155 to 158).

Mental health doesn't divide neatly into sections or chapters; the various issues are totally interrelated. This book includes cross-references to help you find material in different chapters, and includes an index for overarching topics like depression, children's mental health, and violence, that appear in more than one place.

Adapt this information for your community

This book includes discussions of what community-based organizations have done. It also gives practical examples of how individuals experience, get through, and support each other's mental health challenges. We hope you'll find both useful.

One of the prime lessons of community organizing is: Everything is connected. Sometimes as you draw out those interconnections, life can feel overwhelming. Supporting mental health need not feel overwhelming, and we hope this book helps individuals and organizations find and offer support in both small and big ways.

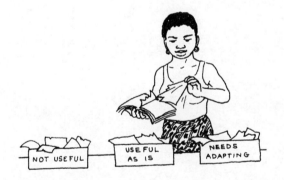

There is no one right way to address mental health and no one strategy that works for everyone. Take the ideas that look most useful and try them out, adapting them along the way to fit your community and situation.

When we share the successful experience of a community group, remember that one of the reasons for their success is that their work is rooted in a specific place, history, and people. Starting where you are and building on your community's strengths will provide you with a rich source of creative and achievable solutions.

We need your help—tell us how to improve this book!

Hesperian's book creation process involves gathering feedback from those with experience—in this case, with community-based approaches to addressing mental health—as well as from anyone using this material in any way in their work. Your frank and constructive criticism and feedback will help make future editions better. Stories from your experiences will expand the variety of issues covered and the richness with which they are discussed. Contact us at MentalHealth@hesperian.org to tell us what you think.

A word on word choices

Hesperian Health Guides believes that language has the power to shape and change hearts and minds. We do our best to use inclusive language that recognizes the value and importance of every individual and community in the struggle to create a more just world. Language changes over time as we create that more inclusive society. Multiple words to describe a condition or group of people are often in use at the same time, and not everyone will choose the same one for themselves or recognize how language has changed at the same time. Understanding the effect of different words and how preferred terms evolve is especially important when describing communities who face persistent injustice. To honor and respect our organizational partners in this book, we have written about them and their work using the words they use on their websites and in their other materials. We hope the language choices found here reflect our common commitment to promoting community mental health.

1 Building community builds mental health

A community is a healthier, happier, and safer place when people feel connected. Knowing that you are not isolated or alone, that there are people who share a similar situation as yours, makes you feel better about yourself and your community.

Connecting with others also leads to more people helping each other out in small ways as well as joining together to fix bigger problems. Starting out can be as simple as gathering to clean up the school yard or creating an event for neighbors to meet. Building community can also include ongoing efforts to end violence, fight discrimination, prevent hunger, and stop evictions. Large or small, any improvement in housing, jobs, schools, and the conditions to lead a dignified life allow people to worry less, and suffer fewer hardships.

Community organizing is mental health work

People may not think of organizing or participating in community activities as mental health promotion work. Yet all these efforts clearly support community mental health—they help people get to know their neighbors better, develop their abilities to change things for the better alongside others, and make the community a more enjoyable, fair, and safe place.

There are many ways to support and grow a stronger community, including:

- Find spaces in urban areas to create parks where children can play, adults and teens can relax and socialize, and groups can gather for tai chi or dancing, or to grow food in community gardens.

- Celebrate culture by holding events with food, music, dance, different types of art and artists, presentations and films, and spiritual practices or rituals.

- Invite and support young people to participate in music, the arts, and sports, and to have time outdoors and in nature.

- Reclaim and celebrate community history by marking or restoring sites with historical meaning, and involving elders to pass that history on to youth. Removing or replacing monuments symbolizing harmful or incomplete ways of telling history is sometimes a first step.

Back to the garden: Domestic workers care for each other

Joining together for mutual support is incredibly powerful. This is especially true for domestic workers because it's not easy to find one another. Domestic workers are nannies, housekeepers, and caregivers each working for one or two employers. Domestic workers are not properly appreciated despite so many in US society depending so much on them. The stressful work, low wages, and long hours make other parts of life difficult too. *Domestic Workers United* (DWU) in New York City was founded to push back against the invisibility and isolation of domestic work, and to help workers know their rights.

DWU members discuss shared challenges and organize to improve working conditions. They show how creating community heals and brings hope, directly improving everyone's mental health and showing the pride and beauty of Caribbean, Latinx, and African cultures.

DWU activities help domestic workers gain power and respect, but the shared sense of community is what helps people get through each day. Members connect over text and meet Saturdays at a local community garden under a giant willow tree to lift up, encourage, and support each other. When someone is facing a tough time, a member tells them: "Come back to the garden."

"Community is each of us and our families. It is our cultural networks, neighborhood networks, and ties to our home countries."

"Community is food: gathering where it's grown, handing out bags of fresh produce, and sharing herbs that heal and foods we prepare with flavors from the islands."

"Community is finding the artist within us, sharing stories, dancing, and joining public theater and writers' workshops. All ways of telling our truth to power."

"We are building a movement. Together, change is possible and feels good!"

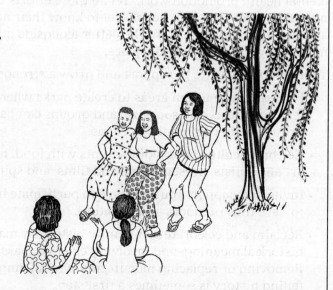

Community connections build power— and mental health

Most of us are part of several communities. Where we live is the most common kind of community. We may or may not know our neighbors well, but we share neighborhood experiences such as breathing polluted air or feeling frustration when public officials do not respond to community needs. Busy streets that are dangerous to cross, fear that people we know will be harmed by violence, and lack of good public transportation to get where we need to go are other examples of problems we may share with neighbors.

Other kinds of communities include families who send their children to the same school, those attending the same place of worship, and your co-workers at your job. Many of us also feel part of communities that share an identity (for instance the same race, ethnicity, language, sexual orientation, health condition), similar values or beliefs (such as religious or political beliefs), or the same problems, interests, hobbies, or talents. While feelings of community connection are often stronger when we can get together in person, connecting online also allows us to create or join communities with others no matter where they live. All types of communities provide opportunities to meet more people, form friendships, and work together on common projects.

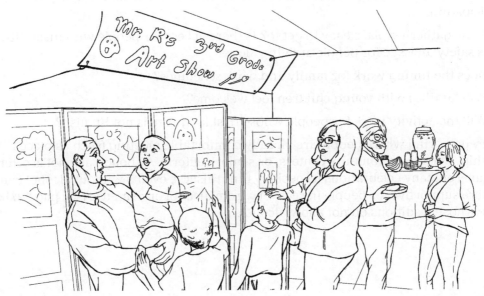

Community involvement is good for mental health. The feeling of belonging you get from connecting with others who share similar ideas, needs, or goals can make you feel joyful, safe, and relieved that you are not alone. It can also be a relief to learn how many of your experiences are shared by others.

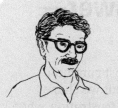

We were upset that hateful graffiti directed at the Muslim community began appearing on walls in our town. We discussed how fear and hate come from people who don't know much about you. We looked at The Islamic Networks Group website for ideas on how to plan a "Know Your Neighbor" get-together. They had sample flyers and step-by-step instructions for a storytelling night, a tea party, and other ideas. We decided to hold a cook-off contest at the school featuring local restaurants that serve Halal food. The students all attended with their families, we played some group games and printed recipes to take home. There is something really basic about eating together that builds trust. It was a fun way to get people to mingle and to learn a little about our Muslim neighbors, their faith, and their food.

When you create community where it wasn't obvious "a community" existed—for example, when you begin working with people from different economic or cultural backgrounds because your kids go to school together—you help overcome what previously seemed to be unbridgeable differences or divisions. Learning about each other's struggles and achievements can help forge shared solidarity and common purpose. The world needs more of this, as does our mental health.

Ideas for bringing people together

Think about how to fully welcome those who will have the most difficulty participating.

- Is the gathering place easy to get to? Is there access for people with disabilities? Is safety an issue for people arriving alone?
- Does the timing work for family and work schedules?
- Will families with young children feel welcome?
- Will the activity work for people whose first language is not English?

Try gathering where people are already comfortable meeting (such as places of worship, schools, community centers, or senior centers). Although alcohol is often available at many celebrations (especially fundraisers), events without alcohol can be more supportive for people in recovery from alcohol or drug use (see page 97) or those whose traditions do not allow alcohol.

Health promoters create and sustain community

Latino Health Access (LHA) in Santa Ana, California, focuses on community participation as the best, most long-lasting way to make communities happier and healthier places. While acting on specific mental health issues, such as supporting people with grief and loss, adjusting to diabetes, overcoming older people's isolation, and creating supports for women facing domestic violence, LHA's activities bring people together to spark community change. This makes everyone feel better about where they live and get along better with their neighbors. Adapting the Latin American *promotor* model of community leaders reaching out and connecting individuals and groups who otherwise might not find each other, the LHA *promotor* becomes a person to turn to in a crisis.

LHA's *promotores* are community members helping other community members make things happen. *Promotores* organize the community for civic participation and political actions that can create or change policy. They organize the community, including young people, to rally for peace within homes and across neighborhoods, advocate for parks and safety, and create healthier environments for all families. *Promotores* help their neighbors access different services, programs, and systems to become more independent, yet the *promotores* always remain a constant, friendly part of people's lives. *Promotores* identify and befriend people who are isolated, advocate alongside them, and offer ongoing support for them and their families.

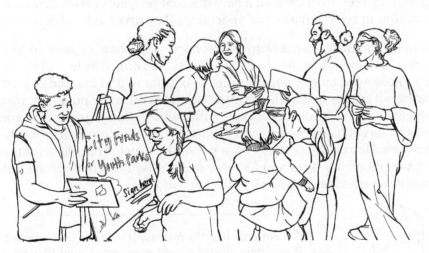

People in the community have learned to believe in the *promotores*. They see how they have consciously and successfully improved their own lives, so they gratefully accept their help as role models and teachers.

Green is life: Detroit urban farming and greenways

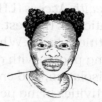

The fact is, people feel better in green space; they respect themselves more. People want to live in a place that has beauty and is healthy. Greening supports that from the ground up.

Our health, including our mental health, suffers in urban spaces without places for children to play, for sports, for families to enjoy time together, or for people to walk, bike, or use wheelchairs or strollers. Growing food in an empty lot, adding plants to a traffic median, and lobbying for bike paths are activities that bring people together twice: first, to pursue a common goal; and second, to encourage even more people to "harvest the fruit" of using the new space.

The Detroit, Michigan, non-profit, *The Greening of Detroit*, started in 1989 with one part-time volunteer. To date, 1,350 local residents have graduated from their workforce development programs, 30,000 youth have participated in year-round programs, and 150,000 trees have been planted. Growing the urban forest and creating skilled green jobs brings positive community change. Since 2016, *Keep Growing Detroit* envisions a city where the majority of fruits and vegetables consumed by Detroiters are grown by residents. By supporting beginner gardeners in becoming engaged community leaders and food entrepreneurs, they have created a network that provides urban growers with opportunities to sell the fruits and vegetables they grow at local markets.

Another organization, the *Detroit Greenways Coalition*, organized to make biking feel safe and attractive. In 2006, the city had only 6 miles of bike lanes. By 2023, there were more than 150 miles of bike lanes and marked shared lanes. Bike paths not only help people get exercise and reduce car pollution, they also get people outdoors. By encouraging cycling and walking, greenways connect people of different backgrounds and promote friendlier, more neighborly communities. Detroit's bike paths have paved the way for regular events such as Thursday-night group rides and Monday-night Slow Rolls that attract hundreds of people of all ages, races, and class backgrounds.

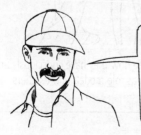

It's not only healthy for people and the environment, but it also gets diverse people mingling in ways they wouldn't otherwise. When people are on foot or on bikes, they're meeting and engaging. That's important in this region. The more people meeting and mingling, the better.

Build support and solidarity

When a group of people facing similar problems comes together to identify the stresses and harms affecting their community, doing something about it is their logical next step.

- Making the harm go away or become less harmful can improve the well-being of group participants and neighbors right away.

- Achieving one change can open the door to other changes and inspire people to think about what might be possible.

Another benefit of taking on a community project is how people themselves change as they get involved in organizing. Even if they lose in the short-term, they win something in the long-term. They develop new relationships, new insights into their own power, and new ideas about what is possible and what is blocking their desired changes. Group action and community organizing build support and solidarity. People grow their strengths as individuals and power as a group by working together.

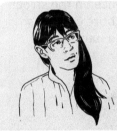

I'd like to think that I will be around to one day see the better world our struggles are trying to create, even though I know change doesn't happen overnight and we are up against deep and historical injustices. But I have a different thought as well: these are struggles that have to be fought. Not because we know we will win them, but because it is the right thing to do.

There is no question that these projects can take a great deal of effort and hard work. Working with others to make change is fulfilling, but long hours, setbacks, and a sense of too-slow progress is usually part of it as well. Often there are no shortcuts to things that take time. Staying in it for the long haul means reminding yourself that lifting up collective mental health ultimately will prevent—as well as repair—many problems people experience as individuals. And an affirming and positive process to get there is part of the cure.

Preventing violence: Start with a street corner

Sometimes a group has to challenge power structures and create alternatives to the way things are. Taking action by being present and strong together can challenge harmful policies and practices and at the same time model how problems affecting a community could be handled differently.

Mothers and Men Against Senseless Killings (MASK) started as a small group of volunteers in a Chicago neighborhood known for high levels of gang violence, police violence, and other problems. The group set out to break the cycle of violence by occupying a central street corner. They wanted a neighborhood where everyone, especially children, could be safe and could flourish.

They started with volunteers bringing chairs and sitting outdoors on the block every evening. The group also began to cook and hand out food to support neighbors, which also got more people to spend more time outside on the street and helped the adults to get to better know each other and connect with young people.

Building relationships with youth and a more constant presence on the street helped to calm problems that arose among young people. Neighbors could also watch out for police, protecting anyone the police might stop and harass.

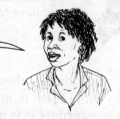

Looking back after years of work, we could pinpoint how change occurred. People began to notice neighbors were watching out for each other, and that was contagious. Now this method of injecting good vibes into troubled areas is catching on in more communities.

MASK has had setbacks along the way—some of their members were lost to the gun violence they work to eradicate. Rather than giving up, they expanded to meet more needs, setting up counseling and guidance for community members. They provide a listening ear for people who need it. And to try to address some of the deeper causes of violence, MASK connects neighbors, especially youth, to city services, educational opportunities, economic support, and professional skills training.

Getting to the roots of problems to improve community mental health

When people right in front of us are showing distress or having a mental health problem, of course we want to help them right away. We focus on them, what they are going through, and what might help them feel better. Some mental health professionals (including social workers, nurses, counselors, religious leaders, and others) skillfully do that time and time again. They help a succession of people heal.

To improve community mental health, we need to make sure people get the person-to-person help they need, and we need to identify and change the conditions that create and worsen mental health challenges for entire groups of people. These conditions may be social, economic, or political, and many started long ago. These deep and ongoing sources of stress and hardship also make it more difficult to recover from hard times, such as a death in the family, a relationship ending, or losing a job or a home.

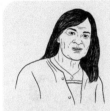

In our work supporting the health of Native Americans, we ask if the person or their parent went through the trauma of being sent to boarding school, a US policy for decades. The resulting loss of cultural ways, forced family separation, and unresolved grief may still impact the mental health of a Native survivor or their child today.

By helping people identify and work to change these underlying conditions, as well as build skills to cope with stresses, community mental health work can strengthen an individual's ability to withstand the impact of the disappointments and even tragedies that happen in life. Community mental health efforts can also strengthen, support, and sustain groups of people when such events disrupt a neighborhood or community.

ACTIVITY But why?

Finding the root causes of mental and physical health problems means looking at the different parts of our lives and the systems that contribute to those problems. The "But why?" discussion technique helps us look deeper and shows how problems, and their eventual solutions, are usually not caused by individual decisions but by larger social issues. Raising awareness of how these affect us can help us organize effective action for change and build resilience in individuals and communities. "But why?" also helps us sift through complex situations to identify smaller parts that are more easily changed.

You can use "But why?" to discuss a specific problem or situation, or you can make up a story that reflects the conditions in your community.

1. Start by describing the situation and asking the group to share their ideas about why it happened. After each answer, ask "But why?" to explore more underlying causes for as long as people keep thinking of reasons.

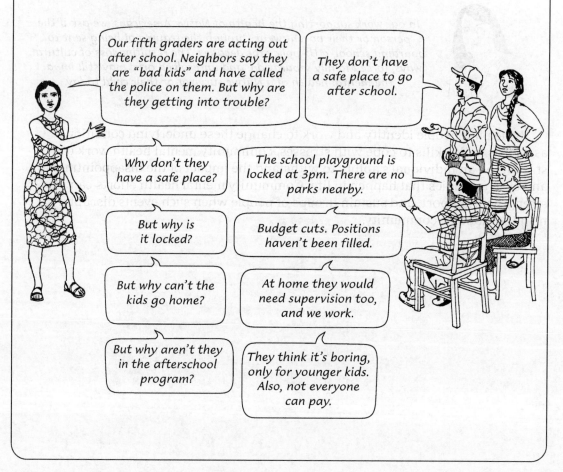

Our fifth graders are acting out after school. Neighbors say they are "bad kids" and have called the police on them. But why are they getting into trouble?

They don't have a safe place to go after school.

Why don't they have a safe place?

The school playground is locked at 3pm. There are no parks nearby.

But why is it locked?

Budget cuts. Positions haven't been filled.

But why can't the kids go home?

At home they would need supervision too, and we work.

But why aren't they in the afterschool program?

They think it's boring, only for younger kids. Also, not everyone can pay.

ACTIVITY   **But why?** *continued*

2. Ask the group to reflect on the many underlying causes they found. Talking about all the causes of a problem can help the group decide which causes are the most important, which causes can change, what are possible solutions and who—both inside and outside the group—can work for those changes.

3. Then ask: What actions can address the causes of the problems?

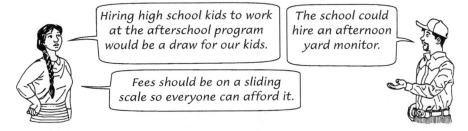

Hiring high school kids to work at the afterschool program would be a draw for our kids.

The school could hire an afternoon yard monitor.

Fees should be on a sliding scale so everyone can afford it.

4. To conclude, help the group come to agreements on which action or actions they will start with, and develop a clear plan for next steps.

This "But why?" technique is also good for looking at successes. It can help you think more deeply about what went well and why, and what that might tell you about planning next steps for the group or working on other problems.

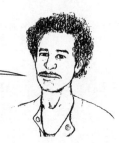

We looked at the neighboring town's popular teen center. Asking "But why?" uncovered what was behind their success: dynamic staff, a variety of sports equipment, and teen leaders promoting it on social media. All strategies we can apply here.

Activism, policies, and programs responding to community issues can prevent as well as cure some of the causes of mental health problems. This is the big picture that is sometimes forgotten or overwhelmed in the face of individual mental health needs. Skill-building to prepare us to support people (including ourselves) going through a hard time will improve our effectiveness in meeting our community's needs and working for change. Recognizing the signs of mental health challenges, paying attention to how we interact with others, and developing listening and de-escalation skills are among the topics examined more deeply in the following 3 chapters.

2 Stresses affect mental health

Common, everyday situations often create stress. This includes everything from a loud, unexpected noise to arguing with someone in your family, to preparing for a test in school, to misplacing your keys. Usually, the stress comes and goes, and we go on. We don't all experience the same moments of stress in our lives, or react the same way to them, but we all experience stress. While extremely stressful situations or terrible events can cause trauma that people often need help addressing (see page 34), mostly, stress is something we "just deal with."

Many people live with ongoing, harmful stresses:

- Working several jobs to get by, having too little income or a lot of debt.

- Abusive or unhappy relationships.

- Challenges related to rough times as a child, or young adult, or for people who had to change countries or move to a new place to find safety.

- Discrimination because of how you look, who you are, or from ideas others have about you. These can be based on race, gender, sexual orientation, disability, body size, customs, language, or other reasons, including mental illness. Discrimination can be direct and dangerous but also can happen in small ways that wear away at you over time.

Stresses come regularly from illness, work, or family life, and for children or young people they often come from school environments and online interactions. Even exciting events, like a new baby or starting a job, can be stressful because they create big changes.

People respond to too much stress in different ways. Some people get angry more easily while others are overcome with worry and doubt. Stress makes it impossible for some people to make decisions, while others are pushed to make snap decisions without thinking them through. People may use alcohol and other drugs to try to lower their stress, which may lead to additional problems.

If you are one of the many people who "just deal with" stress, it can help to identify the methods to beat stress that work best for you. Many people find overcoming a challenge leads to more confidence that they can do it again next time. Helping each other get through stress and stressful times can bring relief, and when group actions or supportive social programs remove some of the stresses altogether, this lightens the load people carry.

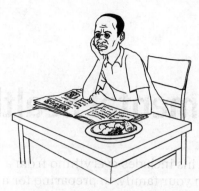

Stresses can take the joy out of life.

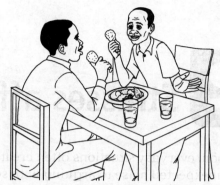

But you don't have to face stress alone.

Stresses affect the body

When stress or fear happens suddenly, you can feel it in your body—your heart beats more quickly and your breathing may change. And then, as the stress fades, you often feel your body relax. Short-term stress is common for everyone and not always a problem. In fact, responding to and getting through stress is often a rewarding part of our emotional health (see "Stress and anxiety are not always harmful," page 33).

When someone is stressed all the time, it can build up and affect them more. Sometimes the stress in our lives doesn't directly affect our thoughts and feelings, but the body shows it is there. Common conditions such as trouble sleeping are often tangled up with stress. Stress can also show up as body aches and pains or illnesses we can't explain another way.

People often get used to stress and don't notice how it is affecting the body, even when the stress is enough to cause harm.

Stresses that continue for a long time (for example, from a high-pressure workplace or an abusive relationship) can cause both mental health challenges, such as anxiety and depression, as well as physical signs, including headaches, lack of energy, and stomach upset or other intestinal problems. Ongoing stress can lead to long-term health problems including high blood pressure and heart disease, diabetes, and problems affecting the immune system. For example, racism and other types of discrimination in the US cause very high rates of stress-related physical problems in Black communities.

What we notice about our bodies holds clues about our emotions and gives us ways to manage them. While our bodies often hold stress, they also often hold the keys to reduce stress—that is why many people consider sports, stretching, walking, dancing, and other physical activity to be "stress busting." There are many techniques to use our own body awareness to reduce stress, including acupressure, finger-holding, reflexology, breathing techniques, and other practices (see examples on pages 21, 31, and 140).

HOW TO   Use finger-holding to manage strong emotions

Techniques involving pressure points, pressing on specific points on the body, can help make people aware of what is happening inside them.

Using finger-holds in challenging moments can bring peace, focus, and calm. This calming can give you time to think of the right response or action to take. Finger-holds can also be used for relaxation with music or before going to sleep, to release the problems of the day and bring peace to body and mind.

You can do this for yourself or you can hold the fingers of someone else who is angry or upset. The finger-holds are helpful for crying children or tantrums. They can also be used with people who are very fearful, anxious, sick, or dying.

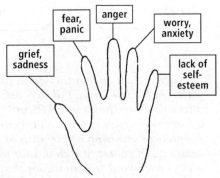

1. Start by wrapping either of your hands around one finger of the opposite hand. Choose one finger to focus on a source of stress, or go through all 10 fingers one at a time. People often focus on each finger being connected to a specific feeling, such as:

- The thumb for sadness or grief

- The index finger for fear or panic

- The middle finger for anger

- The ring finger for worry or anxiety

- The little finger for low self-esteem or trying too hard

2. Hold each finger with a firm touch for at least 1 to 2 minutes and up to 5 minutes. As you hold each finger, you often feel a pulsing sensation.

- Focus on your breath moving in and out of your body and simply feel the feelings instead of thinking about what events or life circumstances caused them.

- Breathe out slowly, releasing the feelings and problems. Imagine the negative feelings draining out of your finger into the earth.

- Breathe in a sense of harmony and healing.

Emotions can be like waves of energy moving through the body and mind. You can make a channel of energy connecting each finger to a particular emotion or part of your body.

Dealing with all the stress

Because it is impossible to completely avoid the things that cause stress, people learn to handle them enough to get through each day. By connecting with others going through similar situations, you can lessen stress by talking it through or by sharing activities such as exercise, meditation, community service, singing, or creative arts. Working with others to change conditions in the community can help people feel better now while also preventing mental health problems by removing or lowering stresses that affect everyone.

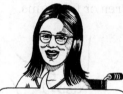

We taught the 4th and 5th graders meditation techniques and have 10 minutes daily of quiet time. The kids now look forward to it.

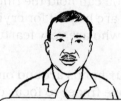

Twice a month I pack grocery bags at the food pantry. I'm not saying it will end my neighbors' poverty, but at least they won't be hungry while we work toward bigger solutions.

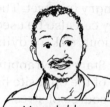

My neighbor and I grew up with the same music. We get together, play our favorite songs, and sing along loudly!

I teach a class on mental health for community health workers from different backgrounds. I always ask: "What do people in your family or culture do when things are difficult?" Many people mention tea—brewing tea or inviting someone to join them for tea. Another common response is practices involving water, such as relaxing in water, bathing, or foot-washing. Of course, watch out for practices that may cause harm, but always ask about the traditions that work for people already. We often hear new ideas we each want to try!

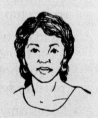

Food, exercise, friends, and nature

You hear about it a lot and it's true: nutritious food, exercise and movement, being with other people, spending time outdoors, and getting enough sleep all help prevent many physical and mental health difficulties as well as help us manage them better. This is why so many community groups and health programs make these a focus.

HOW TO   Pick a health habit to try out or do more of

Is there something you already like to do that you know is good for you? For example, walking in the neighborhood, eating fresh fruit, drinking more water, getting a little extra sleep, spending time outside—even when it's cloudy and especially if the day is sunny. Think of this as your secret weapon to lessen stress, change what's on your mind, and make you stronger. To start, make your goal small enough that you know you will achieve it. Doing one thing well usually makes people see they can continue or even do more of it.

Doing it with others can make it more fun. Maybe you can make a pact with another person or a group to check in about how each of you are doing with your goals. Not all goals will work out, but if you find something that feels good and is doable, you will see that you can change things in your life. Try different ideas.

- Walk 2 or 3 times a week, even if it isn't very far. Try some errands on foot, or you can get off the bus or park the car so you walk a little extra each day.

- Get together to cook or eat with someone, trying a new food or recipe.

- Drink more water—plain water, water with lemon, or unsweetened herbal tea—with meals and during the day.

- Agree with a friend that you'll each go to sleep 15 minutes earlier than normal, or, if your phone is keeping you from sleeping, agree to put your phone in a different room a few nights per week.

If starting a new health habit on your own or with a friend isn't working, see if a community or senior center offers workshops or classes—often free or low cost—and choose something that sounds interesting or fun to try out. Try to interest a friend in going too.

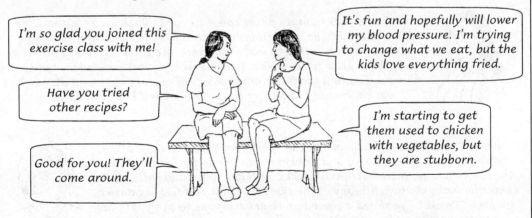

I'm so glad you joined this exercise class with me!

It's fun and hopefully will lower my blood pressure. I'm trying to change what we eat, but the kids love everything fried.

Have you tried other recipes?

I'm starting to get them used to chicken with vegetables, but they are stubborn.

Good for you! They'll come around.

Help others think about their goals by asking more about them. Almost no one likes being told what to do but it is OK to encourage someone to come up with their own ideas of what could work.

To change our health habits, we often need more than personal strength and initiative—we need communities where having healthy habits is not so difficult! Think about what keeps people in your community from living a more healthy life and what could make it easier.

- If the water in school cafeterias tasted good and no soda was sold, would more kids fill up their water bottles?
- If parks and bike and walking paths were kept clear of trash and felt safe to use, would more people use them?
- If there was a community garden, affordable neighborhood farmers' market, or community meal program, would people eat healthier food?
- Are there historical or cultural traditions that used to bring people together which could be revived?

Stress makes diabetes, high blood pressure, and other chronic illnesses worse. And living with these conditions can cause more stress. I reverse this negative loop that creates stress by treating my diabetes, including eating well. That helps with the diabetes but also improves my energy level and mood.

Our city park has always funded a summer outdoor yoga class. This year we mixed it up by finding community members who do other movement— hip hop dance, belly dancing, tai chi, and "bring your baby" stretching. More people started to come and the teachers we hired were happy more people could try out their classes.

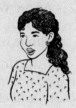

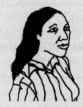

It took us a year to make a tule canoe as our Indigenous ancestors used to. We learned to be in relationship with tule by harvesting it, drying it, and then working with it to make the canoe. We came together every few months to pray, to remember Indigenous technical knowledge, and to share stories and songs. We made plenty of mistakes to laugh at, but it was enormously satisfying to see our finished boat could float!

Where I teach, the high school kids talk a lot about their anxiety, often while eating cookies or chips and drinking soda or energy drinks! We got the school to offer more nutritious snacks, with less sugar and caffeine. For kids who make the switch, many of the signs that look and feel like anxiety go away. The kids organized a campaign to get everyone to carry refillable water bottles and the school to improve the water fountain filters.

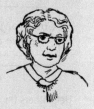

Being there for people

Along with improving where we live, we can create communities in which people are aware of others' needs and offer more emotional support. You don't need special training to feel concern for another person and start a conversation. Although a private, quiet place to talk might be ideal, any available time or place is probably OK. Ask if they have a moment to take a walk or join you for a cup of coffee or tea. Sitting together on a playground bench while they watch their children may be an opportunity to check in a little, even when their life is very busy.

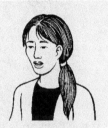

I knew my neighbor has family in a country going through violent times, though I didn't know much about it. One day I asked after her family. She looked so sad and then relieved—saying she is terribly worried but few people know this is on her mind all the time. Now we exchange a few words whenever we see each other, and I pay more attention to the news reports about her country.

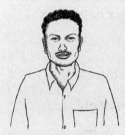

When worried about someone—maybe we think they drink too much alcohol—it is tempting to speak about it directly. But if the person doesn't experience it as a problem, then either it isn't a problem or, as long as they don't see it as a problem, they won't want to deal with it. I test the waters first. For example: "I've noticed you seem to stop for a drink after work before coming to our meetings. Is that something you want to talk about?" If they react negatively, be ready to let it go. You have planted a seed and maybe they will come back to you about it in the future.

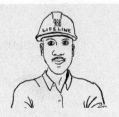

Construction workers die from suicide 5 times more than from jobsite accidents. Our tough-guy worker culture means that if you are hurting, you hide it from everyone—at home and at work. I always remind my crew: "It's okay to not be okay" and tell them to look out for each other. We need to make it okay to ask how people are and okay to answer honestly when you are asked.

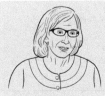

I worried that my elderly neighbor was lonely during the day. I started giving her a ride to the neighborhood church on my way to work twice a week. She now sings in their choir and helps maintain their garden. It reopened her world and she always thanks me for it.

HOW TO   **Offer emotional support**

If someone lets you know they are going through a rough time or if you think they are, it's common to not know what to do or say. The good news is that just being there for someone can be extremely helpful. In fact, for some people just knowing that someone is thinking about them, someone cares, someone will visit now and then, can make a real difference in their mental well-being.

- Once you feel ready to listen, check if the person is OK with you asking.

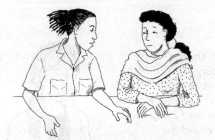

"I've been wanting to know how you are, is it OK if I ask?"

"If you are OK talking about it, tell me how it's been going for you lately."

If the person is not ready, mention you're available if they change their mind.

- Listen more than you talk and let the person talk freely. Use questions that get the person talking instead of questions where the answer is "yes" or "no."

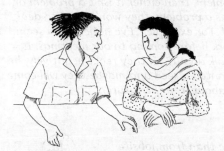

"What did you do then?"

"Tell me more about that."

"And how did that feel?"

- Offer empathy and reassurance. Be affirming when appropriate.

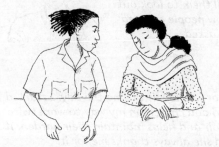

"That must have been very difficult."

"I can see it was a hard situation where you did your best."

"Sounds like you learned a lot from that."

HOW TO   **Offer emotional support** *(continued)*

- Stay calm and be patient.

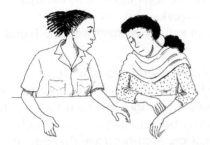

"Take your time. We are not in a hurry."

"We can just be quiet with these feelings for a minute."

"Thank you for sharing that."

- Do not make assumptions or minimize what they are feeling or experiencing. Choose words that show you are open to and not judging what they share.

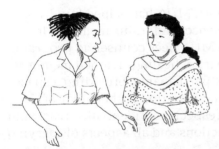

"I appreciate that you can share that with me."

"That isn't something I know much about, so I'll learn from whatever you can explain about it."

"I am sorry to hear people keep telling you, 'It's no big deal.' I can hear that it was a big deal."

- Focus on not giving advice. It is tempting to think you can help people fix their problems, but they are the only ones who can decide how to handle their situation. It can take a lot of restraint not to give them solutions! Instead, ask about what seems to work for them already and what they want to do about their situation. Offer to help find more information only if you know you will follow through. Remember, sometimes listening is enough.

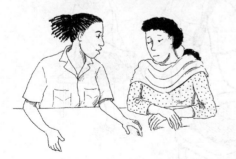

"What are you thinking you want to do?"

"Say more about what worked for you last time this happened."

"That's a great idea. Do you know what is stopping you from trying that?"

"Do you want help looking into some options for that?"

"You don't have to decide right now. This is something you can think about."

Peer counselors strengthen ties and build resilience

Finding and training people who have had similar experiences or are from a specific community to help others with similar backgrounds or situations is called peer counseling. Peer counseling often works best because the counselors understand the experiences of community members and are trusted differently than outside professionals.

Mujeres Unidas y Activas (MUA) is a California-based organization of immigrant Latina and Indigenous women workers. Members speak Spanish but many also speak Mam, a Guatemalan indigenous language. MUA's mission is to increase their members' personal and community power, and use civic-political participation to achieve social and economic justice. Members are directly in charge of MUA advocacy campaigns, and each person gains skills by lobbying, calling representatives, giving testimony, and taking to the streets to stand up for workplace health and safety and women's rights.

MUA's practice is centered on mutual support. MUA has helped hundreds of women get out of situations of domestic violence, and trains members to gain leadership and legal advocacy skills. The MUA peer counseling program, *Clínicas del Alma*, builds leadership and is a part of healing. Trained members are available to support others, especially new participants, providing a space for each woman to speak freely about what is on her mind without fear of judgment. The organization is a space where respect, confidentiality, trust, and empowerment are woven into everyday interactions and all aspects of carrying out the work.

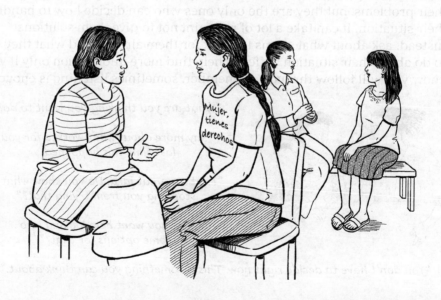

ACTIVITY Practice being a good listener

If your group members are new to each other, talk about how to take in other people's experiences while keeping your heart and mind as open as possible.

It can take practice to set aside our own ideas and to listen without assuming we know more than what we are being told. This is especially true when people have different experiences due to where and how they grew up or live now.

Practice listening. The group divides into pairs. One person talks about a topic for 5 to 10 minutes, picking from a few prompts. For example: "Talk about something that is challenging in your life," or: "Describe an issue the community is facing." Their partner listens without commenting except to encourage the speaker to say more. As a listener, show you are paying attention with your expressions and by facing the speaker.

Then the two people switch roles. When they are finished, they consider how well it worked. They ask each other questions like:

- *What did I do that made you feel I was listening?*
- *Did anything make you feel I wasn't listening closely enough?*
- *When it was your turn to listen, what was hard about it?*
- *If you wanted to start responding while you were listening, how did you stop yourself?*

Then have a general group discussion about ways to best show listening and concern. Discuss how listening sometimes includes talking, such as asking questions, sharing experiences, and saying, "Thank you for sharing that," or "I understand."

Remember, when you do not understand something, you can ask the person to explain more.

Variation. To have the group reflect on the natural tendency to want to give advice, have the listener give lots of advice about the problem presented, even to the point of being pushy. When the partners talk about it afterwards, they can say what it felt like to get advice. Then try again, focusing on giving support, not advice.

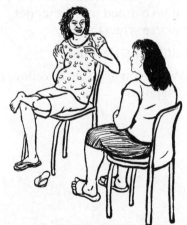

Anxiety

Everyone feels nervous or worried from time to time. When these feelings are caused by a specific situation that can be fixed—perhaps your rent and electricity bill are due, but then your paycheck arrives in time—they usually go away soon afterwards.

For situations that you know make you anxious, learning how to make yourself feel calm can help (see "Regain calm," page 31). If the feelings continue or happen too frequently, you may need help to identify and address what is causing the worry and anxiety. This could be planning ahead (for example, to avoid anxiety about being late for appointments because buses run behind schedule, you could plan to leave earlier) or coming up with a new strategy (for example, to worry less about your child's safety, you could organize with other parents so all the children on your block walk home together). Where the cause of concern is related to larger injustices or problems that make you worry for yourself or others, don't stay alone with it. As a first step, find and talk with others who are experiencing the same situation or feelings.

Feeling worried all the time

If you stay worried or always fear the worst will happen, and there is no specific situation that is causing your worries, then you may need help from someone who has experience counseling people about anxiety.

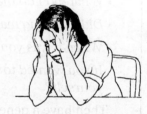

Constant worry may come with other signs:

- feeling tense, restless, or nervous

- difficulty thinking clearly

- sweating, headaches, muscle aches, stomach aches, or unexplained pains that get worse when upset

> My brother is so afraid of germs that he no longer leaves home and rarely sees people. We are talking with him—does this feel like a problem to him? If he wants to get out more, what would make that easier?

- difficulty sleeping

When you are able to relieve or control the anxiety, often these other signs lessen or disappear.

HOW TO   Regain calm: Find what works for you

There is no one strategy that calms everyone and stops anxiety, fear, panic, or anger from taking over. In fact, some people who feel anxious find that deep breathing makes them more anxious! Try different techniques and decide which work best for you. Some people count beads on a necklace, squeeze a ball, stroke something textured, smell a soothing scent, press their fingers on the body's pressure points, or use finger-holds (see page 21). Spend time with pets if that gives comfort or draw on your traditions or faith practices (prayers, mantras) if these help you. Practice calming exercises in group settings and with children. Learning what others find calming can add ideas to your own list.

Breathing. Deep breathing and breathing exercises help a lot of people calm down quickly. It can be as simple as breathing out a little longer than breathing in: breathe in for 4 seconds, then breathe out for 6 seconds. (See page 140 for another breathing exercise.)

Distraction. If helping someone, ask them to describe: 5 things they can see, 4 things they can hear, 3 things they can touch, 2 things they can smell, and 1 thing they can taste. Doing something to refocus your thoughts can help the body settle down more quickly.

Visualization. Choose a calming image— gentle waves lapping a sandy beach, towering trees filtering sunlight in a quiet woods, a kitten with soft fur snuggled on your lap—and practice keeping it in your mind. Then bring that image to mind in moments of stress by closing your eyes and concentrating on it. Longer visualization stories can also move your mind to a calmer state. For example, picture yourself beside a beautiful river where you are slowly dropping leaves or petals into the current. Imagine they are worries or problems as you watch the river carry them away.

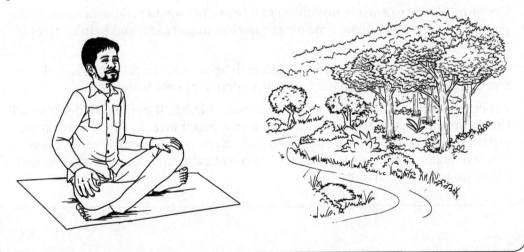

Panic attacks

A panic attack is a severe kind of anxiety. Panic attacks happen suddenly and can last from several minutes up to a half an hour. In addition to the signs of anxiety (see page 30), you may feel your heart pounding, have chest pain, have difficulty breathing, and feel that something terrible is about to happen.

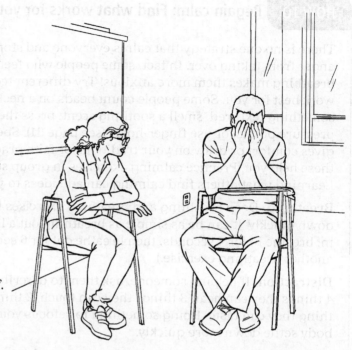

If you have repeat panic attacks, practice slow breathing at other times so you are prepared to use it when needed to calm yourself. Similar to using medicine to lower a fever, slow breathing can help you stop a panic attack but it does not resolve the problem that caused it.

HOW TO   **Help someone during a panic attack**

Help the person regain control of their breathing. Help them focus on deep, slow breaths, inhaling through the nose and exhaling out of the mouth.

Counting slowly to 4 while breathing can help a person breathe more slowly. Be patient—it might take some time for the person to feel calm and gain control of breathing.

Another way to interrupt a panic attack is to hold an ice pack, a package of frozen food, or ice cubes in the hand, or to drink ice cold water.

Especially when a person is older or in poor health, it can be difficult to tell the difference between a panic attack and a heart attack. Often heart attacks are triggered by physical exertion, and their chest pains intensify more slowly and last longer than a panic attack. If you're not sure, do not take a chance: call 911 or go to a hospital immediately.

Stress and anxiety are not always harmful

A student may have trouble sleeping before a test, a worker may feel overwhelmed by a deadline, an athlete may worry before a race, and a community leader may feel her heart pounding before speaking at a big meeting. Sometimes stress and anxiety help us prepare for important tasks. These feelings can help us focus on a goal, make the time to plan ahead, or work especially hard. Knowing how and why our bodies react in these situations can help you use stressful feelings to your benefit. This can help you feel more ready for the situation you are facing.

Find what works for you. Everyone has worries and fears, and how we respond to these is different. Something that is a problem for one person may not be a problem for someone else. The biggest indication of whether a person needs help for their anxiety is how much it affects their daily life.

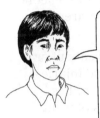

My teen daughter is often fearful and needs support to try new things. But she knows that her hesitation also keeps her from taking risks like her friends do.

I was always anxious and superstitious that my worries might cause something bad to happen, which led to problems for my family and my work. In my church, we have a group where I practice how to talk about, face, and then "put away" my worries so they don't affect me so much.

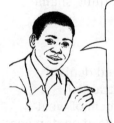

The only way to get to my new job is by driving. I took lessons and got my license but am so fearful it makes me feel sick before work. A counselor is helping me because I just have to overcome this.

My youngest child is different from his sisters. He is very organized and neat at home and at school. He worries more about germs and remembers to wash his hands. But these habits work well for him: he does well in school and rarely gets sick.

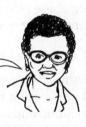

Part of finding what works for you is accepting how people's brains work differently (this is called "neurodiversity") and celebrating its benefits, such as "outside the box" problem-solving. Where neurodiversity is experienced as a disability, society should do a better job of meeting people where they are. For example, specific sensitivities—to light, noise, new people, or crowds—interfere less with enjoying daily life when there is awareness and support. A shrill-sounding school bell may make a few kids especially anxious but by changing to a softer sound, all the school children will benefit.

Trauma

Sometimes stressful experiences are so overwhelming they cause trauma. Trauma is an emotional or physical response to a terrible event a person saw or went through in the past or is going through now that feels life-threatening to them or others. Examples include being in an accident, abuse in the family, violence, rape, torture, displacement, and large-scale disasters. Trauma can follow:

- a single incident, like a dog bite.
- a horrific event affecting many people, like a mass shooting.
- ongoing or past events, like growing up in a violent home.

Trauma can make a person feel unsafe, insecure, helpless, and unable to trust the world or the people around them, either sometimes or all the time. Trauma recovery can take a long time. An old traumatic experience can still be a problem for someone, especially if they never had help healing. Trauma that happened to one's parents or ancestors can also have lasting impact.

We may know survivors of trauma, even if it is not something they talk about or we are aware of. This includes adults affected by abuse or other childhood injuries, sometimes before they were old enough to understand (see "Violence in families," page 76). A person may remember feeling terror without recalling details of what happened. Or people will remember the events but not remember the feeling of terror, which can make it harder for them to understand their continuing problems. Sometimes traumatic situations are still occurring, and people fear that talking about it could cause them or others further harm. Some people who experienced violence or abuse also were abusive toward others. This can lead to confusion, guilt, shame, anger, fear, and other painful feelings.

Common signs of trauma

Immediately after a traumatic event, people often experience shock and denial. Longer-term reactions include unpredictable emotions, flashbacks, strained relationships, avoiding people, and avoiding anything that reminds them of what happened. They may have depression and physical problems such as head or stomach aches, nausea, difficulty concentrating, nightmares or insomnia, hopelessness, and feeling like nothing matters. These reactions can be part of more lasting effects from trauma known as post-traumatic stress disorder (PTSD, see page 55).

People who have experienced trauma may be jumpy or constantly alert to danger, may feel irritated or angry, and may always have the trauma on their mind.

Reacting to trauma, the mind may try to protect itself by separating body, mind, and emotions, usually experienced all together. The person may remember feeling nothing during the traumatic event, or feel "like I was outside of myself watching it happen from a mile away." The separation between feelings and body can become a habit. It can cause numbness as another reaction to trauma.

Support people who have experienced trauma

Ways to support people following trauma include:

Provide a sense of safety. People can have a hard time recovering their sense of safety even if the trauma is over. The body stays in the state of responding to danger, so the person doesn't feel safe. Help them feel more comfortable. For instance, if they don't feel safe talking with you in a room with the door closed, ask what would feel OK, like a bench in a quiet corner of a park where others are around.

Would you like to sit here or prefer we walk outside while we talk?

Show you are trustworthy. When people have experienced trauma, they may be cautious with others, always on edge, and fearful of attack or betrayal. You can show you can be trusted by being predictable and by not hiding anything. For example, be on time, avoid promising something unrealistic, do exactly what you say you will do, and clearly explain why you are doing things and why you are asking certain questions.

I know you count on the food bank groceries. We are closing for a week, so if you want, let's see which other food program might work for you next week.

Give a sense of control. In a traumatic situation, people experience a loss of control. Help people regain control by giving them choices, big and small. Have them decide if, when, and where they talk with you, participate in decision-making, and know what will happen next.

Welcome to today's 2-hour legal aid workshop. Staff will look after the kids in the art and play room, but children can also stay with parents during the workshop if you all prefer. We'll have a lunch break at noon.

Take it seriously. People who have experienced trauma may feel isolated or out of sync with the rest of the world. Be aware of the conditions that continue to create danger and cause trauma in people's lives, and show you take them seriously. By openly recognizing that racism, for example, targets people for violence or unequal treatment, you can demonstrate that your support is not dependent on them accepting the conditions that caused their trauma.

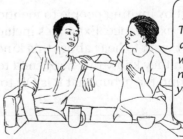

I hear you. The way you describe the white doctor not believing you, that is a problem.

Group activities to help people living with trauma

For some people, connecting with others who have faced similar types of trauma can be helpful in feeling less alone with their experiences. (Chapter 8, "Support groups," includes ideas about how to set up and run support groups.) Here are some ideas for group activities.

Help people share their experience

When a trauma occurs, people often feel that it shouldn't be talked about. They may feel shame, as if there was something wrong with them that brought it on, or that they are damaged or tainted by what happened. Sometimes they feel no one wants to hear about such a horrible thing, which increases their isolation.

ACTIVITY **Speak the unspeakable**

Facilitating a support group for people who have experienced trauma can bring up a lot for the group and the facilitators. Talk with others who facilitate such groups to decide whether you have the resources and experience to take this on.

When setting up a support group, provide clear information ahead of time about what to expect. That way, people can decide if they are ready to share some parts of what they are dealing with and to hear about other people's traumatic experiences. Follow suggestions on pages 133 to 134 for starting support groups, including establishing group agreements of how information will be kept private and other ways to help people feel comfortable.

If you know everyone feels ready to connect with others with similar experiences, introduce the idea of "the unspeakable." Part of what makes a trauma a trauma is how alone people often feel, as though what happened makes them not belong, that no one could understand or wants to hear about it. For some people, writing, drawing, working with clay, or other forms of expression can work better than talking, so make art materials available during the group. Let people know they can share a drawing or something they've written instead of talking. Or they can pass if they aren't ready.

1. Start by inviting people to mention what can make it hard to talk about their experience. Examples include: "I don't want to think about it," "People don't want to hear about this kind of thing," "People look at you differently when they know this happened to you," "It was worse than words can say." Remind the group that it is OK to choose not to speak.

ACTIVITY   Speak the unspeakable *(continued)*

2. Share the idea that part of feeling better after experiences like this is finding ways to connect with others—being seen and heard by others—rather than staying all alone with it. Ask the group to name the things that others can do to convey that they are listening/paying attention. Examples include: "Don't look directly at me, but don't act like you are ignoring me either," "Take a moment to think before you respond."

3. Give people a set time (perhaps 5 minutes) to think about the experience that brings them into the group. You might say: "This group is for people who have experienced gun violence in our communities. Take 5 minutes to think, write, or draw on your own about your experience with gun violence."

4. Explain they can choose to talk, read out loud something they wrote, or show a drawing. Suggest they focus on a small piece because it is common when talking about trauma to get caught up and feel like it is happening all over again. Let the group know that there will be a time limit and each person will have the same amount of time to share. As always, people can pass if they don't want to share.

5. Invite people who feel ready to take turns sharing part of their experience, talk, read aloud something they wrote, or show a drawing. After a person has shared, with the group showing they have been listening, ask if they felt heard and how it felt to share before the next person begins. Remind people to avoid commenting on what others share.

6. When everyone who wants to has shared, invite the group to reflect on what people are thinking or feeling after the sharing, or something they learned or appreciated about listening to others. Be clear that people are not being asked to talk about anyone's specific experiences or to give advice.

Activities like these can bring up hard-to-manage feelings. Get group agreement at the beginning to support one another and have a plan to provide additional mental health support if needed. If you are co-facilitating with others, make time to debrief and support each other following a group meeting. If you are facilitating by yourself, plan how you will debrief after the meeting and have support.

Creating the more complete story

Traumatic events harm a person's way of understanding the world. They might experience this as a spiritual crisis or the end of everything familiar: "Nothing makes sense anymore." Someone who feels as if senseless, horrible things can happen at any time may question if life is worth living.

Creating a fuller story of what happened that puts it in the context of a person's broader, complex life can be part of healing. This may include "speaking the unspeakable" (see pages 36 to 37) as a first step. It may also help to "tell a story" that makes the trauma just one part of a person's life and remind them that their life includes a past, a present, and a future. A group can come together to create stories that provide connection and empowerment through artistic or documentary expression.

Digital stories. *Voices to End FGM/C* has connected with groups in the US and other countries to support survivors of female genital mutilation or cutting. They use storytelling and media production so survivors can tell their own stories on their own terms. The stories are made into short videos and used for social justice advocacy to prevent female genital cutting practices.

Creative storytelling. *NAKA Dance Theater* supports healing circles with immigrant domestic workers through theater, movement, textile art, collage, and other arts. One group produced a theater piece and a color zine to reflect on their experiences of forced migration, violence, and injustice in the workplace. The zine doubled as a journal for future participants by including questions for reflection and blank pages where people could write or draw their own stories.

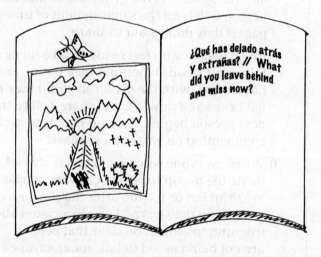

¿Qué has dejado atrás y extrañas? // What did you leave behind and miss now?

Help resolve feelings of blame

One consequence of experiencing trauma is that people may feel betrayed by their loved ones (or others on whom they depended) for "letting" this happen to them, even if a part of them knows it is more complicated than that. Adults may feel let down by partners, government officials, or neighbors, and children may feel let down by caretakers who did not protect them. Adults, in turn, may feel shame for not having been able to protect a child or a spouse.

Helping people talk about these feelings or explore them through art can be important to healing, to making space for understanding that what happened was not their fault. It can also help people rebuild and strengthen their "protective shields"—the real abilities that we have to protect ourselves and others under ordinary, non-traumatic circumstances.

ACTIVITY   Repair the protective shield

This activity can be used to help someone while they think about the person they feel let them down. Or it can be done with the two people involved, such as a parent and child. Start by talking about how hard this activity can be and why it is important. Both sides are hard: feeling let down by a loved one and feeling that we failed someone we love. If you are doing this with a parent and child, help the parent anticipate that it can be hard to hear what the child expresses but that it is important to hear them out completely. Explain that this is part of an ongoing process, not something that can be healed quickly.

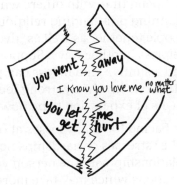

1. Invite the person to draw a shield shape.

2. Guide the person to talk about specific things that happened that made it feel like the shield was not working, for example, "You didn't come when I called you," "You left me alone," "You didn't stop the fire from burning down our house." With each statement, make a rip or use scissors to make a cut in the shield.

3. Invite them to look at the broken shield and talk about the thoughts or feelings that come up.

4. Then invite them to list things that represent protection and patch the broken shield. Use masking tape with words written on it or images cut out of magazines showing healing or protection. For example, write, "You come and hold me when I'm scared at night" or add a picture of a watchdog.

As you look at the broken/repaired shield together, invite them to talk about their thoughts and feelings.

Grief and loss

Grief is our response to loss. Loss is always a part of life, and processing loss through grieving is essential to mental health. It is common to feel overwhelmed with grief or go through a long or difficult grieving process with:

- the death or approaching death of someone close.
- the death of someone in the community or a respected person, whether or not there was a personal relationship.
- the end of a relationship, a divorce, loss of a job, being forced to move or losing a home, having a serious or ongoing illness, or adjusting to a disability.
- tragedies that affect many people at once, including violence, displacement, and disasters.

Although all of us will experience grief, different people will show and experience grief in many different ways. Grief has no single pattern or timeline. People in your family or community who have experienced the same loss may go through it very differently. Even after time has passed and it seems the hardest part is over, intense feelings may return. Ups and downs can continue for a long time. As feelings gradually ease, it becomes more possible to live with the loss as life moves on.

Support for grieving

After a loss, paying attention to your eating, exercise, and rest, and accepting support from others can help you get through the first weeks and months.

Spend time with others who are grieving the same loss or who can relate to yours. Planning or attending religious or other rituals for burial or remembering can bring people together as well as give them something specific to do when they may feel helpless in other ways. Support groups (see page 131) with participants who have had a similar kind of loss can provide a place to work through feelings. As with other situations involving strong feelings, many people find writing, music, art, or other forms of expression to be powerful ways to process grief and loss.

Facing too many losses at once or losing someone when you are experiencing other stresses or hardships needs even more attention. If you had a difficult relationship with the person you lost, you may be working through a bigger mix of emotions which may take more time.

When supporting another person, you can accompany them as they go through pain, but your job is not to take away the pain or tell them when it will go away. Accept their feelings and their timeline. You can be a comforting presence; listen if they want that, and find out if there are tasks or responsibilities you can take off their plate.

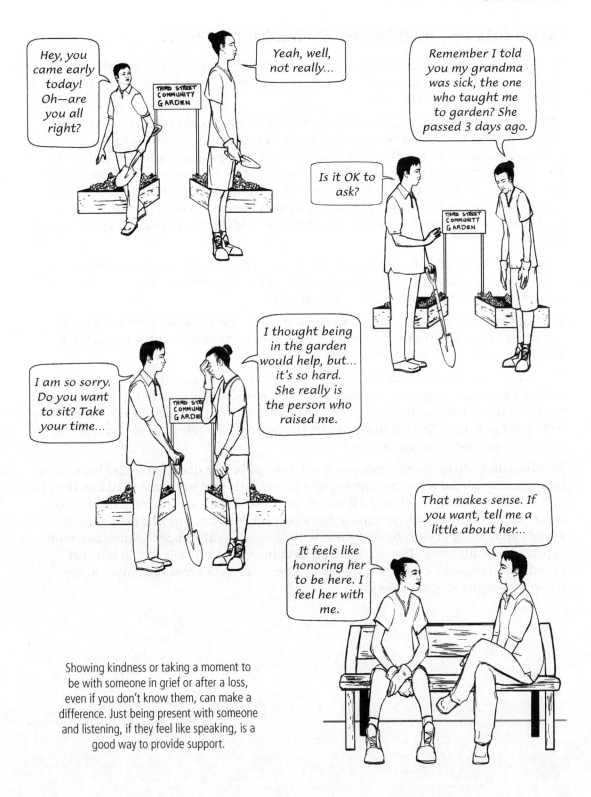

Showing kindness or taking a moment to be with someone in grief or after a loss, even if you don't know them, can make a difference. Just being present with someone and listening, if they feel like speaking, is a good way to provide support.

When loss can lead to mental health problems

A blocked grieving process can lead to mental health challenges, especially depression. Emotional difficulties can be created or made worse by ideas about when and how much grief is OK to feel.

Mismatched timeline. People often say or act like you should be "over it" or should "move on" when that does not match where you are. Though calming for some, routine caretaking or meeting other family expectations and household tasks can feel overwhelming when trying to grieve. Society, the workplace, or religious rituals may expect you to grieve at a different pace than your feelings are developing. You may have no or too little time off before you are expected to return to work, or be expected to participate in observances that schedule certain feelings to specific time periods.

Conflicted feelings. Having difficult or mixed feelings about the person before they died, such as being angry at them or feeling guilty you didn't do more for them, can make it harder to feel settled about their death.

Hiding grief. Stigma and shame can block the grieving process. For example, if you lose a loved one to a drug overdose, you may feel shame or anger about their substance use, and this can block your grief.

Avoiding grief. Using alcohol or other substances to manage emotional pain, working too many hours, or relying on television, video games, or online scrolling to avoid thinking about the loss can displace the grieving process. While distraction from grief may be helpful at times, it can also prevent the release that you will feel by going through necessary grieving.

Needing more help. Sometimes, the hard feelings of loss don't get better even after time passes. Painful emotions remain severe and interfere too much with life. If signs of depression (see pages 45 and 54) make you think someone is not recovering from loss or is not able to move through a grieving process even with the help of their friends and family, try to connect them with mental health support. Some common experiences with grief—for example, not sleeping or eating well, losing interest in regular activities—do not always mean a person has depression, however, even though the signs may look the same.

Helping children with loss

Children grieve differently than adults, in ways related to their age. Young children can know when they or someone else in their household is very ill, or when someone has died. They may not understand all the actions and feelings of people around them, but they know when something is wrong.

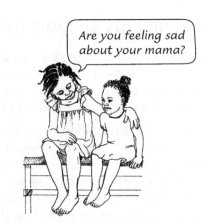

Are you feeling sad about your mama?

When someone is very ill or, following an accident or after someone has died, everyone in the family feels distress, including the children. A child may respond by misbehaving, wetting the bed, not eating, not speaking, or acting younger than their age. Children do not decide to do these things; they just have no other ways to show their distress. Helping them learn how to process their feelings will help them throughout their entire life (see pages 85 to 86).

Children who lose someone close to them need loving attention, patience, and support as they grieve and find ways to go on with their lives.

Ways to prepare a child for loss

Many families avoid talking with children about serious illness, death, divorce, and other serious situations because they think that not hearing about such problems protects them. But not talking with children may leave them afraid of what is happening, alone with their fears, and shocked later if there is a death or someone close to them is no longer there.

Talking with a child about these topics can be difficult, but helping children prepare to face a difficult situation or death in the family, and then talking with them about it afterwards, is very important. How a child reacts to upsetting news often depends on how the adults are handling it. When adults appear strong and calm, children often respond that way too.

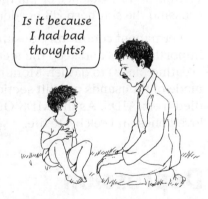

Is it because I had bad thoughts?

Allow children to ask questions. Answer their questions honestly, giving them truthful information they can understand based on their age and ability to understand. Share small amounts of information over time as the child adjusts to what they see happening. Let them know any feeling they have is OK to have and OK to tell you about. For example, a child might reveal their worry that it was their behavior that caused a person's illness or accident, and they need to be reassured that is not true. Show them understanding and affection, praise them when they do something well, spend time with them, and give them the attention all children need.

Community support for grieving

Helpful traditions. Ask about and offer ways to connect people to others who share their traditions about death and grief. Especially when someone has moved recently, or is from another country, they may want to reconnect with cultural traditions but do not know where to find others who share them.

Create meaning. Many people find comfort in organizing to prevent others from going through what they did. People may share powerful testimonies, work to change policies, or raise money for a larger cause when their loss is related to a specific illness, type of violence, or accident. Joining with others in common cause creates bonds and emotional support. Creating resources and support networks can bring comfort in knowing that the next person needing the same information will benefit from your experience.

Commemoration and memory. Religious and spiritual practices help many people find comfort or meaning after a loss. People can also create their own spaces or moments in which to remember and honor loved ones. This can be as simple as lighting a candle or finding a beautiful spot for quiet reflection. These occasions can be very personal, shared only by family, or more public. The Mexican and Central American tradition of creating altars to express both celebration and sadness on the yearly Day of the Dead has inspired many beautiful and meaningful altars to individuals and groups, for example, people who were victims of gun violence or partner violence or died crossing the southern US border.

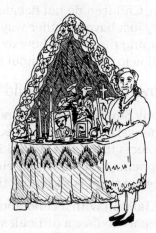

Permanent community-designed monuments, plaques, parks, and gardens mark important sites and keep the memory of people or group histories alive as well as creating places to gather. Monuments can be mobile too. The *AIDS Memorial Quilt* is made of thousands of quilt sections sewn by families and loved ones of people who died from AIDS. As the AIDS Quilt travels, it brings people together to remember loved ones and celebrate life.

Depression

It is natural to feel sad at different times—when a friend or family member is very ill or dies, when you lose a job, when a relationship or marriage ends unhappily, or after a serious event or tragedy. In these situations, sadness can last for days or weeks, or it can come and go (see "Grief and loss," page 40).

Depression, however, is different than sadness that follows a difficult event or from feeling distressed by the state of the world. Depression is when feelings that include sadness, hopelessness, or numbness are present all the time.

You may have depression if sadness lasts for weeks, if you feel useless or hopeless, or if you don't want to leave the house or even get out of bed. Depression sometimes doesn't feel like sadness at all, but more like being in a fog where nothing seems important. Depression is a serious medical condition that affects a person's life, ability to make decisions, and ability to function.

A person with any of these signs that do not go away may have depression. Even if it is not depression, they will need help and support:

- feeling sad most of the time, feeling hopeless, or being numb to feelings
- sleeping too much or too little
- difficulty thinking clearly
- feeling guilty
- feeling like crying or crying frequently for no apparent reason
- loss of interest in activities that a person used to enjoy, including eating, spending time with others, and sex
- lack of energy for daily activities

Severe depression (see page 54) is when depression lasts a long time and strongly interferes with a person's ability to function. If someone has been talking to you or others a lot about death or suicide, then take them seriously. Try to talk with them to see what kind of help they think they need (see page 65).

Some people are embarrassed to be depressed and do not want anyone to know how badly they feel. But depression is an illness, not a sign of weakness, and is no one's fault. Let them know that you are OK with them as they are and that you believe there are things that could help them feel better that they have a right to access.

Help for someone with depression

Although it is hard to believe while in the midst of it, a person experiencing depression can "get their life back." This is true even when depression is a long-term condition that will likely stay a part of their life. Finding the right support and treatment is key.

Talk therapy. For some people, coping with or healing from depression is helped by counseling or other types of talk therapy, being part of a support group, or working in social change groups.

Movement or touch. Some people are also helped by addressing how mental health is felt in the body. Techniques include focusing on the body during talk therapy and touch therapies that provide insights or release.

Medicines called anti-depressants are sometimes combined with the other types of therapy, especially if symptoms are severe. Figuring out if medicines or other treatments will work and which best suits a person is a process. Having an ongoing connection with the same health worker or team of people allows changes to be made over time to adjust the treatment, medicine, or dose. Medicines do not work for everyone, and the use of medicines can create problems too. It is important to remember: the social conditions that cause many mental health problems will not be fixed by medicines, but by social change. (See more about medicines on page 50.)

Asking even a trusted person for help can be very hard for a person with depression because the condition itself often makes people feel unable to do anything. This makes support from others even more important. It can be a big relief to find someone who knows what depression is like, who can offer accompaniment, and who can help find the services available for people with depression.

Preventing mental distress in LGBTQ+ youth

LGBTQ+ youth in the US are more likely to experience depression and other mental health problems, a situation made worse without support from family and friends. Teachers and school staff may notice challenges faced by students in the process of defining their gender identity and sexuality. School-based efforts, such as Genders & Sexualities Alliances clubs, can provide support, protect students from mental health stressors, and prevent some young people from developing depression. It takes courage, but these and other efforts (see page 121) are especially important when LGBTQ+ communities are under attack.

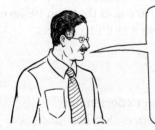

Build a supportive network of adults at your school so that students have safe places to be. Let the students determine if they want to be activists or if they want to put all their energy toward supporting each other. Even if attendance is low, keep publicizing the meetings. Just announcing it in the weekly school bulletin can be enough to let an LGBTQ+-identifying kid know there are people out there who care.

A place to just be yourself. *Color Splash Out* is a camp program in Texas where young people have fun and also get support as they think about their gender identity. The affordable program is run by counselors with a variety of gender identities who help kids feel OK about being exactly who they are, even if they don't have a name for it yet. Kids appreciate being nurtured in a way they can carry back to other parts of their lives: "Having friends here who get me makes school tolerable when I'm back home."

Pushing back on what pushes people into depression

Conditions that make depression more likely include:

- living with constant stress or worrying about meeting basic needs, such as access to housing, health care, safety, and food.
- experiencing something terrible or that feels catastrophic, such as major loss or severe illness.

Community efforts to lower everyone's stress and insecurity (the focus of Chapter 1, "Building community builds mental health") will improve conditions and make it more likely everyone has someone or a network of people they can turn to when they need support. Strong friendships, knowing your neighbors, and quality workplace relationships are important parts of what keeps depression away. The community-building we can do to push back against isolation and disconnectedness makes a big difference.

3 Serious mental illness

Some people experience mental health challenges serious enough to require more intense treatment and support. Because people have very different personal situations and varied ways of handling emotions, there is no clear line between what is serious or severe and what is just challenging. Nevertheless, there are similarities in what people experience as severe. In general, severe mental illness means people are not able to carry out routine functions of everyday life or to safely care for themselves.

Examples of serious mental health illnesses include:

- severe depression
- bipolar disorder, when someone alternates between being very depressed and very keyed-up (manic)
- post-traumatic stress disorder (PTSD), when past traumatic events cause a person's body to be in a constant state of alert or numbness
- psychosis, a disconnection from one's surroundings and being in a different reality than others experience
- schizophrenia, a type of psychosis, which interferes with the perception of reality, the organization of thoughts, and the ability to have a full range of feelings

Our society's lack of openness about mental health creates stigma and discrimination for people with mental illness. Some people won't talk about it or even use the words "mental illness." This does not help.

A basic understanding of mental illness can help you connect someone who needs support to a doctor, counselor, or community clinic, and to provide support yourself. Unfortunately, health systems in the US make getting respectful, helpful, and affordable care very difficult, if not impossible. Options are so limited that the choice can be between insufficient care or being locked up. Psychiatric drugs may work well for some people but create even more problems for others. Health insurance may sometimes cover costs of mental health treatment, but there can be long waiting lists and limited treatment options. People of color often find mental health providers to be culturally inappropriate and insensitive to the stress and trauma caused by racism. Too often, these barriers prevent us from getting the care we really need and instead we just accept what we can get.

The chances of getting quality and long-term care for mental health in the US are so bad that medical professionals, news media, and even politicians are seeing the situation as a crisis and calling for action. Progress so far is due to the many dedicated individuals and organizations working to reduce the inequalities and conditions that cause mental health problems and limit treatment. This momentum opens a space for you and your community to mobilize to address the most pressing mental health needs and help construct this movement for change.

Treatment with medicines

When they work well, psychiatric medicines can calm people, make them feel less anxiety, allow them to concentrate and feel productive, and ease distress in a variety of ways. But like other medicines, sometimes they have too strong of an effect, side effects causing new problems, or even the opposite effect of what is intended. Some people believe that these medicines are the only thing that allows them to lead a "normal" life. Others find the medicines harmful, saying that they deny them access to their feelings and their genuine self.

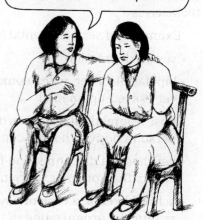

I know you don't like taking your meds. But when you don't take them, you tell me that it's hard to communicate and to concentrate. Are you OK with me going to the clinic with you to ask about other options?

Medicines are sometimes used as a quick fix instead of full-time accompaniment, intensive talk therapy, or community building among people with mental illness. If integrating different approaches was better supported through funding, policies, and medical education, such treatments could lessen the use of psychiatric medicines and their unwanted effects. But when other treatment approaches lack social supports and are unavailable or unaffordable, patients and their families and friends are left with very difficult decisions.

When a mental health provider prescribes a medicine and the person agrees to use it, it may take some time to find the right medicine and best dose. It can also take time for the person to get used to the medicine's effects. Which medicines are available or a person's needs can change over time. Many people find it helpful to involve a close friend or relative while trying out medicines. This other person can check in about how the medicines are working, what side effects are happening, and what to do if a medicine does not work well.

Using psychiatric medicines does not change a person's need for a supportive community, regular meals, exercise, and stable housing. If more people could live without worrying about these basic needs, it would prevent at least some serious mental health illness. Addressing them should always be part of helping people heal and have stability.

Community awareness and support

Mental illness is a community issue, especially because of stigma, discrimination, exclusion, and the lack of understanding that leads to people with mental health concerns being penalized, isolated, mocked, or feared. Similar to other types of disabilities, as a society, we need to make more room for people with mental illness to participate fully in social life, make contributions, and live in the least restrictive way that is safe.

Story of the new neighbor

A new neighbor moved into a house in a small rural town. He spent a lot of time on his front porch, so many people greeted him and exchanged small talk. Neighbors commented that he was a little mysterious, but perfectly nice. Then one night, he took a hammer and broke the windows of the cars parked near his house.

Someone called the police and he was arrested. Some of the neighbors whose cars had been damaged attended the court proceedings a few weeks later. They learned that their new neighbor had bipolar disorder and had stopped taking his medication, which led to his drastic change in behavior.

The man's parents, who lived a few hours away, arrived to support their son. The parents had hoped that quiet, small-town life would be a good environment for him and help provide the stability he needed to stay on his medications. The townspeople decided to give their new neighbor a second chance and talked with him about how they could work together to prevent this from happening again.

He said he would be OK with having regular check-ins with two neighbors to see how he was doing. He agreed to give them contact information for his parents and his doctor. Understanding more about his situation and finding out what he found helpful and unhelpful, community members set the stage for ongoing support that would hopefully prevent another crisis, avoid the police, and keep him out of jail.

By talking about and preparing for mental health challenges as part of everyday life, we show anyone experiencing them that they are not alone, they will not be discriminated against, and they don't have to hide their situation. This means establishing new habits in our communities and workplaces to make them more welcoming to people with mental health challenges—which at some point or another, includes all of us.

At work we discussed all the common phrases we use casually that are related to mental health, such as "crazy," "nuts," "that's mental," or "he's losing his mind." Along with building awareness about hurtful language related to gender or race, also think about the impact of words you hear and say related to mental health.

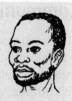

There are probably people in your life, community, or workplace who have, or previously had, a serious mental illness. They may be managing their illness so well that unless they tell you, you would have no way of knowing.

If someone in your workplace or community lets you know they have a mental health condition, you can ask if this is something the person wants others to be aware of, and if it causes them any barriers to full participation. Without assuming that they need help, invite them to let you know if there are any supports or accommodations that would be helpful.

Community-based art to challenge stigma and create connections

Stigma in US society makes living with mental illness so much harder than need be. The multi-year *NYC Mural Arts Project* brought the experiences of people living with mental health conditions to New York City neighborhood walls while creating connections. Each mural involved a group process putting people with mental illness at the center of lively art-making workshops with friends, family, and neighbors. Each workshop series was hosted by a community-based group—a mix of schools, job readiness programs, public housing resident associations, and others.

To come up with mural themes, community sessions were led by a mural artist and one or more Mental Health Peer Support Specialists—people living with mental health challenges trained to support others in the same situation. They discussed community challenges, needs, and desires to craft the mural's message while forging new relationships among participants. The result was people working side by side to break down stereotypes around mental illness, and neighborhood-enhancing murals that continue to raise awareness.

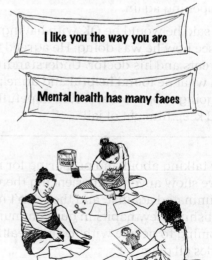

I like you the way you are

Mental health has many faces

Noticing signs of mental illness

Being aware of the signs of serious mental illness can help you respond if someone needs help. The more that people get the good, respectful treatment they need, the better the condition will be managed. As is true for all of us, isolation and added stress make things worse. Finding ways to maintain connectedness for the person going through serious mental health difficulties is essential.

Warning signs

Signs of serious mental illness can be similar to those of common and less severe mental health challenges (for example, see "Depression," page 44). It is less worrisome when a person's behavior changes only for a short time or has a clear explanation—such as difficulty sleeping when under extra stress, or feeling deep sadness following the death of a loved one. But if changes alarm you, or if they continue or get worse over time, it could be more serious. Even when people do not talk about what is going on, you may notice changes in how they act, things they say, or just that they seem "off." Signs include:

- Seeming especially down or showing persistent sadness for two weeks or more.
- Feeling tired all the time or without energy to carry out daily activities.
- Avoiding interactions with people, cutting off relationships, or suddenly spending a lot of time alone.
- Saying they feel lonely, without purpose, overwhelmed, ashamed, or hopeless.
- Outbursts of anger or extreme irritability. In children, frequent or extreme emotional outbursts.
- Changes in eating habits, loss of weight, not taking care of themselves as they usually do.
- Difficulty sleeping or having nightmares.
- Using more alcohol or drugs than usual.
- Frequent headaches, stomachaches, or unexplained aches and pains.
- Changes in school or work performance, difficulty concentrating.
- Avoiding or missing school, work, or other usual activities.
- A notable backsliding in skills for children. For example, a child who used the toilet now has frequent accidents, a child who showed independence becomes very clingy, or a child who was talking no longer uses words.
- Drastic changes in mood, behavior, or personality.
- Hurting oneself or talking about it. Saying they want to escape or wish they were dead.

Signs are different for each person and not everyone with one or two of these signs needs medical help. But showing multiple signs or signs that continue over time is a reason to talk to the person and be aware of what might be going on with them. If a person is thinking about or mentions suicide, take them seriously. Speak with them directly about this (see page 65) and connect them to help (see the list of hotlines and other help lines on page 155).

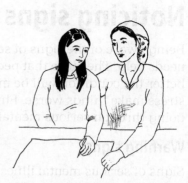

Severe depression

Depression (see page 44) is considered severe based on how long the person has had it and how much it interferes with their functioning. The most important thing for someone struggling with severe depression is for them stay connected, to not feel alone. Make it clear that you are comfortable being with people who are feeling low, that you are interested in their experience, and that they are not a burden when they share their situation with you. Ask what help and support they have now, and what they have found helpful in the past. Ask specifically about medications—are they starting, restarting, or changing medications, either prescribed or self-treating. Using medicines does not always affect depression as hoped, as quickly as hoped, or in a predictable way. To better manage, people taking medicine for depression may benefit from an ongoing relationship with a mental health provider, or at least from checking in about their medications.

A common experience with depression is feeling unable to do anything at all, including something that might lessen the depression, such as exercise or group activities. This can become a vicious cycle. A support group where people share experiences and provide moral support to one another can help break the cycle and make a big difference.

Mania

Mania means being very keyed-up. A person who is manic may feel extremely happy, talk fast, move fast, not sleep, start big projects, make rash decisions, drive too fast, or spend a lot of money.

A person in a manic state can be so caught up in the experience that it is almost impossible to interrupt them when speaking, slow them down, or get them to reflect on their actions. They may believe they are super-important or on a special mission. Mania usually feels good, so people don't want it to end, but it can cause people to do harmful things.

If you see someone becoming manic, stay calm and work to stay connected with them. Listening techniques (described on pages 26 to 27) may be helpful. If the person is about to do something important—like quit their job or make a major purchase, without much thought or consideration of the longer-term consequences —don't argue about whether the idea is good or bad. Instead, encourage them to delay and take some time to think it over. Get in touch with people who know the person well and share your observations about their behavior, preferably with the person present and involved in the conversation. If the person knows they have bipolar disorder or another condition related to mania, perhaps they can check with their health care providers about medications. If this is a new experience for them, perhaps you can help them get an evaluation.

People who have had mania in the past can learn to identify their early warning signs, such as difficulty sleeping, racing thoughts, or a hard time focusing. They can arrange for support when they notice these signs developing and limit the negative effects of their mania.

Post-traumatic stress disorder (PTSD)

PTSD is a severe response to trauma (see page 34) following one or a series of terrible events or situations. Instead of the person feeling better over time, their emotional and physical reactions continue and are severe enough that it becomes hard for them to function. Signs of PTSD can include a person reliving the traumatic experiences in their mind (flashbacks) while awake or at night, interrupting sleep. Other signs are feeling numb or hopeless, severe levels of anxiety (see page 30), being very watchful and always on alert for danger, and overreacting when startled. When responses intensify or continue for months or years and limit people in their everyday lives, PTSD is one way to describe this set of effects of long-term trauma.

While these are common and expected reactions to surviving or witnessing violence or other traumatic situations, finding the right kind of support after the event can help someone heal without developing the difficult and debilitating symptoms of PTSD. Helping someone feel emotionally safe (see pages 35 to 36) is important as well as not pushing them to talk if they don't want to. Make sure they have control over as many decisions as possible.

Supporting someone with PTSD often involves talk therapy, peer and other social support, integrative therapies, and the many traditional cultural strategies that help someone ground themselves and reset their body and mind (see examples on pages 21, 31, and 140). Talk therapies that help can include those focused on what is felt in the body (somatic experiencing), thoughts while paying attention to a back-and-forth movement or sound (EMDR), and new skills to help deal with the traumatic memories (different types of trauma-focused cognitive behavioral therapy/CBT). Psychiatric drugs work for some people, and recent research shows that psychedelic drugs (including MDMA, LSD, and others), given under trained guidance, can help some people with PTSD.

Service dogs help people with PTSD. Companion or service dogs have proven helpful to people with PTSD because, in addition to being affectionate and comforting, they are trained to create a physical buffer and be alert to surroundings in ways that provide reassurance to their human partner. They also can sound the alarm to others if the person has a crisis.

Many non-profit organizations support people with PTSD to obtain, care for, and benefit from a service dog companion. *Canine Support Teams* has a Prison Pup Program that teaches incarcerated women and men to train dogs to support a person with PTSD or another disability. The trauma relief for the person doing the training and gaining the skills to enable post-incarceration employment as a dog trainer are added benefits to the aid that each dog will provide to someone with PTSD.

Psychosis

Psychosis means losing touch with the reality shared by most people. People with psychosis may not be able to make decisions or act as they normally would because the world they are experiencing has changed. They may have hallucinations: hearing voices or sounds that others do not, or seeing, feeling, tasting, or smelling things that are not there. Psychosis can also cause delusions, such as a false belief that they are being persecuted, on a special mission, or being controlled by outside forces. Psychosis can dramatically change thinking, emotions, and behaviors and will disrupt a person's life, making it difficult to initiate or maintain relationships, care for themselves or others, work, or carry out other usual activities. Psychosis is very distressing to experience. It is also very hard to watch someone you know go through it.

Common signs of psychosis:

- **Changes in emotion and motivation.** These can include depression, anxiety, irritability, being suspicious, acting without emotion or showing emotions that are out of place, changes in appetite, and changes in energy.
- **Changes in thinking and perception.** These can include difficulties with concentration or paying attention, the feeling that they or others around them have changed or are acting very differently, a change in or absence of the senses (smell, sound, or color).
- **Changes in behavior.** These can include severe problems getting enough sleep, social withdrawal or isolation, and difficulty carrying out regular activities related to work, family, and other common settings.

HOW TO   Communicate with a person experiencing psychosis

It can be hard to communicate with a person experiencing psychosis because the two of you are not experiencing the same reality. They may not be aware that you find their behavior unusual. With a person showing signs of psychosis:

Use caution and remain calm. While keeping yourself safe, do what you can to help them feel safe talking with you. Do not stand too close or over them. Do not touch them without permission. Speak calmly and carefully, using common, ordinary language. (See "Your safety matters," on page 59 and other communication tips on pages 62 to 63.)

Ask what they believe is happening. Use listening techniques (see pages 26 to 27) and take care not to show judgment or tell them what to do. Ask if they are experiencing something that troubles them, if they notice changes in how they are feeling, or what they are thinking about.

Don't argue. If they are speaking with you about a hallucination or delusion, do not argue with them about it or deny that it is happening. Acknowledge that what they are experiencing is real to them without confirming or denying what they are seeing or feeling. You can say: "I accept that you hear someone giving you those instructions."

Seek help. Try to get in touch with people who know and are trusted by the person. Share what you saw the person doing or saying, preferably with the person present and involved in the conversation. If the person has a condition like schizophrenia that can involve psychosis, ask the person which friends and family may know about their experiences with medications or have permission to talk to their health care provider.
If this is a new experience for them, perhaps you can help them get an evaluation and care. Avoid involving the police, especially when there is no emergency.

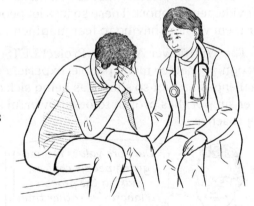

The chapter about helping people in crisis begins on page 59. It includes information about mental health crisis programs that can provide alternatives to involving the police.

Peer mental health support: People who have been there

Integrating peer support into mental health care is remarkably successful. People facing mental health challenges are more likely to trust, listen to, and learn from another person who has faced those same challenges. Because they have "been there" themselves and are committed to not holding power over the person, peer support workers have proven better at connecting with people who often feel isolated and distant from traditional professionals.

In the US, several peer support programs highlight the unique empathy from someone with lived experiences with mental illness, offering a type of mental health care that is culturally and socially relevant and accessible.

Project LETS is a US grassroots organization led by and for folks with lived experience of madness, disability, and trauma, and people who are neurodivergent (meaning their minds work in ways that others think unusual, despite this being very common). The project's Peer Mental Health Advocates work one-on-one with people unable or unwilling to access professional help, as well as people who do have a therapist or psychiatrist but are in need of more support.

The *Wildflower Alliance* has for decades promoted, given trainings for, and been a provider of peer support. Its Western Massachusetts community centers welcome people—without appointments or paperwork—to be with others, participate in community activities, find a support group, or talk one-on-one. Wildflower's Afiya Peer Respite House also provides up to a week of housing (a private bedroom) on short notice when a person needs a place to step away from their living situation with access to peer support 24 hours a day. Online support groups and community discussion through the social platform Discord also provide peer support. These spaces let people share openly whatever is going on for them without having to fear judgment, unwanted advice, or coercion.

The Wildflower Alliance, Project LETS, and other peer support networks recognize that for many people, experiences with severe mental health challenges are not so simple as being sick or being recovered. For some people, peer support has proven to be a powerful alternative to traditional medical approaches.

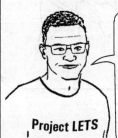

Our core values include giving people choices, making the process collaborative rather than telling people what to do, and making the peer relationships mutual and equal.

Project LETS

Our peer-run respite house strives to provide a space in which each person can find the balance and support needed to turn a difficult time into a learning and growth opportunity.

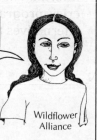

Wildflower Alliance

4 People in crisis

When your community knows you as an activist, health worker, community leader, or involved neighbor, people turn to you for all kinds of support. Sometimes a person may be going through something that feels beyond what you can handle. Even if you plan to connect the person to a mental health professional, you may need to respond to a crisis or emergency by actively providing some direct help right away. This chapter discusses how to prepare in advance for crisis, how to de-escalate and calm a situation, and how to communicate with someone in crisis. Whether acting to prevent a situation from getting worse or facing what is already more clearly a crisis, the priority is always your own safety.

Your safety matters

Always be aware of your surroundings and use the way you move and speak to help calm (de-escalate) the situation (see page 62):

- Stay close enough to a person so they can easily hear you, but out of their reach. There is no way to know if being close to them could make things worse for them or if they could become violent.

- If they have something that could be used as a weapon, try to move yourself and others away until help arrives. Request that they put it down. For example: "I am afraid you holding that makes all of us less safe. Would you be willing to put it down while we talk?" (See "Every crisis is different," page 64.)

- If you are inside, position yourself so the person is not between you and the exit. Make sure exits are not blocked.

- Make sure someone knows where you are and, if necessary, will go to get help.

Consider physical health problems

When someone behaves unusually aggressively or strangely, they may be showing signs of a physical health emergency. You may not be able to get an answer from them directly, but you can ask friends or family with them if there is anything in their health history or current situation that might explain their behavior. Check if they wear a medical ID bracelet. Poisoning or medication overdose, drug use (especially methamphetamine), brain injury or stroke, a diabetic emergency, and serious blood infection (sepsis) can all cause signs that look like mental health emergencies.

Prepare for crises

Reading resources like this one, organizing or joining a training, and using role-plays with scenarios matching your setting, are all ways to gain experience and gain confidence you will know what to do. Also, anyone in a crisis situation will want a trusted person to be aware of what is happening. Plan ahead so your

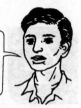

What is a crisis? A crisis is what the person says it is.

communication with a friend or co-worker will be efficient in a moment of crisis. If possible, coordinate with another person to address the situation together, or have one person intervene while the other goes for help.

Preparing for crises also means thinking ahead to know your limits. If you are not OK with the possibility of helping someone in crisis, or only in certain circumstances, know where to turn to for support and who can step in if there is an emergency.

Another way to be ready is to know what mental health and other related resources are available. Keep a reference sheet on hand that includes names and contact information for mental health professionals, women's centers, non-English language support, peer-support networks, suicide-prevention hotlines, and other resources. If you work with an organization, you may already have or want to create procedures to follow in case of mental health emergencies.

Find out if there are alternatives to the police. Many cities are creating non-violent, non-police emergency services to respond to mental health crises. Instead of police, trained mental health workers are sent when someone calls 911 needing this type of help. Some cities also create a different number specifically for mental health emergencies. Find out if your 911 line or other hotlines or peer support lines in your area notify the police and for what scenarios.

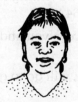

Once you decide which services or people are best to call during a crisis, add them to the Contacts on your phone.

Suicide prevention hotlines. A national suicide prevention line was launched in the US in 2022. You can access it by calling or texting 988. It was also designed to avoid police involvement, though incidents including threats to others might lead to the police being notified. Community-based mental health organizations are monitoring the effectiveness of this new resource. Whether 988 is the best choice for help in your area probably depends on what services are available.

Peer support lines. Peer support lines and other types of "warmlines" are a way to talk or text with a trained peer counselor or professional mental health worker, helping prevent a person's problems from turning into a crisis. *Warmline.org* maintains a list of programs by state. Local clinics and programs may offer warmlines too, and often take calls from everyone, not just people in their region.

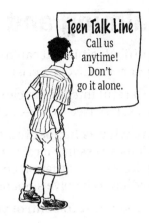

Teen Talk Line
Call us anytime! Don't go it alone.

Hotlines or peer support lines are often established for specific situations, such as domestic violence or drug or alcohol addiction. There are also support lines for people with specific identities or experiences, so they don't have to start from zero explaining themselves. For example, *Trans Lifeline* is run by and for transgender people, and the *Veterans Crisis Line* is for those who served in the military. **Hotlines and warmlines mentioned in this book are listed on page 155.**

Helping someone in crisis

Usually a mental health crisis occurs when something overwhelms a person's regular ways of processing information. What you see as extreme behavior or a strange reaction may be for them a logical response to what they are experiencing. And for them, commonly used words and body language may feel like threats.

I only wanted to help...

A woman was standing on the sidewalk of a busy city street screaming, "Fire! Fire!" and pointing in front of her—where there was no fire. A well-meaning passerby approached the woman, gently touched her back, and said: "Calm down. There is no fire. You are perfectly safe." The frightened woman bolted into traffic. Fortunately, she was not hit by a car.

The woman was having a psychotic experience. The danger she felt was real, although the fire was not. Without meaning to, the passerby who wanted to calm her instead increased her feelings of danger. This was made worse by:

- touching her without permission.
- contradicting her version of reality.

It might have been more helpful to ask the woman calmly, from a distance, if there was a way to help. Also, it may have been possible to make the area around her safer, perhaps by directing people walking nearby to give her plenty of room. *The rest of this chapter has suggestions for communicating with someone in a mental health crisis and other ways to help calm a situation.*

Calming and de-escalating a situation

A difficult situation can quickly change for the worse, but skillful and compassionate support can avoid a crisis.

Careful interaction can calm a tense situation. While remaining conscious of your own safety (see "Your safety matters," page 59):

Note what is happening with the other person, especially if there are signs of serious stress like a raised voice, clenched fist, or confusion. This may be when you realize a calm situation could get worse, leading you to take more safety measures or deciding to involve someone with more experience.

Do your best to control your own physical responses:

- Concentrate on sounding calm and not raising your voice.
- Do not touch the person without their permission and avoid towering over them.
- Keep space between you. If you move, do so slowly.
- Keep your stance relaxed and your expressions as neutral as possible.

Listen carefully, show concern, and offer options as you communicate with someone in crisis (see page 63).

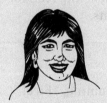

I work in a drop-in site offering different support services to people who use drugs. It helps to pace the interaction and cue what comes next: "We're about to wrap up," "Now that we're done, I'll walk you to the door," "Let me offer you some snacks on the way out." The key is to read people's body language, listen carefully, and be prepared if someone acts unpredictably.

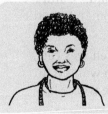

Be calm and patient, and most importantly, open and honest. The person in crisis needs to be able to rely on someone who is not going to be unpredictable or devious. Make them feel safe and supported by you.

HOW TO Communicate with someone in crisis

Your interactions with a person experiencing a mental health crisis can calm the emergency or make it more intense. A central goal of crisis communication is to be as natural and present as possible for the person in crisis. People often respond positively to confidence, calmness, and comfort. Stay aware of your safety (see page 59) and control your body language and tone of voice (page 62).

1. Accept what the person says about their feelings or what they see. Do not downplay or deny what is real for them. For example, do not say: "It isn't so bad," or insist: "You are safe," to someone yelling they are in danger from something you can't see (see the example on page 61).

2. Point out things they are doing in their body to show you are paying attention to them and their feelings: "I notice you are breathing hard." "Your hands are shaking." "You seem to be sweating a lot."

3. Affirm the person by showing your concern. Recognize what they are feeling: "I hear you—you feel very afraid."

4. Ask if there is something or someone that could help them now or has helped in the past. Affirm any practical ideas they mention and help them achieve them if you can (give food or water, call someone they want to talk to, or get other things they may want).

5. Helping people in crisis feel a sense of power and be able to make choices is important. Even small decisions can feel like reclaiming a bit of control over their lives: ask if they would like water or tea, or if they want to sit or stand.

6. If they identify specific things contributing to the crisis, offer concrete actions that might help. For example, if they say: "I am going to lose custody of my child," you might say, "There are resources to help parents and children stay together. We can make a phone call together now if you are OK with that."

7. Do not try to control them unnecessarily. Do not make them sit down if they want to pace, do not make them talk if they want to stay silent.

8. Encourage conversation and communication, but do not force any topics. Say: "We can talk about that later, if you want."

9. Do not use guilt or threats.

10. Do not make promises you cannot keep, such as you will keep secret any ideas they express about hurting themselves or others.

These skills can be practiced in advance by using role plays to imagine and act out different situations.

Every crisis is different

The way you respond to and support someone experiencing a mental health crisis depends on the circumstances. But in every case, stay aware of your safety (see page 59) and consider getting help, especially from those skilled in de-escalating crises (see page 62) and avoiding the police (see page 60) .

If someone is putting themselves or others in danger with their actions, for example: driving while intoxicated, acting violently at a peaceful protest, or throwing objects where there are other people:

- Ask them to slow down or suggest a different course.
- Act to prevent the danger, for example: find an alternate driver who is sober, help other protesters re-route around them, move others out of the room.

If someone seems out of touch with reality and physically unsafe:

- Ask if there is any way you can help them.
- Act to make the environment around them safer by removing objects that could hurt them.
- Tell them you are worried about their health and safety, and ask if you can connect them with someone who can help get what they need to be healthy and safe right now. (Also see "How to communicate with a person experiencing psychosis," page 57.)

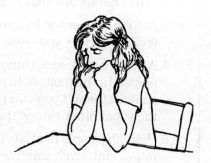

If someone says or shows they are going to physically harm you:

- Get out of the way as much as possible, creating a safe distance between you or perhaps removing yourself entirely.
- If it seems safe, say: "Let's keep talking about this. We can figure this out without anybody getting hurt."
- If they back off from threatening physical harm, follow the guidance about "How to communicate with someone in crisis" (see page 63).

If someone says or shows they are going to physically harm someone else:

- It may be easier and safer for you to remove other people from the situation than to try to move the person in crisis.
- Follow the guidance about "How to communicate with someone in crisis" (see page 63).
- If it seems safe, say: "Let's keep talking about this. We can figure this out without anybody getting hurt."
- You might say: "I'm worried things will get worse if you hurt them. Let's find a way to make things better instead."

- Help them make a plan to stay away from the person they want to hurt, perhaps by staying in the presence of another person who could be a calming influence.
- If you know the person they are threatening to hurt, consider letting the person know what is happening or reaching out to another person who can help.
- Consider getting help, especially from those skillful at de-escalating crises (see page 62) and avoiding the police (see page 60).

If someone says they are considering suicide, or you suspect they are:

- Take them seriously.
- Ask directly, for example, "Are you having thoughts of ending your life?" or "Are you thinking about killing yourself?" or "Are you considering suicide?"
- Show concern but not alarm.
- Be aware that people in crisis may feel ambivalent about suicide. Focus your words to support the part of the person that wants to live, while not ignoring or downplaying the part of them that wants to die.
- Suicide crises are often time-limited. Your goal is to get the person the immediate help they need to get through the crisis and make it to a different state where they can get longer-term help.
- Be collaborative and honest. Say, for example, "I think it is important for you to connect with someone at the clinic about how you are feeling and what might help. Would you be willing to ride over there with me?"
- Although it is important to remain calm and present, rather than convey fear or alarm, you do not have to help the person all by yourself. Talk with them for a while about what they are experiencing, and then say: "I am worried about your safety, and I feel it is important for others who care about you to know you are feeling this way. Can we call your sister to help us think this through?" Or "I am worried about your safety and I would like us to call a hotline together so someone with more experience can help us think it through."

After a crisis

Whether the crisis was resolved successfully or not, it will have an effect on you. Make sure to talk about what happened with someone you feel comfortable with so you get support for the impact the crisis had on you. Also, talk with others about anything you or others could do to help the person or people involved as a follow-up now that the crisis has passed. Discuss with others how the root causes of the crisis might be addressed to prevent similar situations from occurring in the future and how to advocate for the changes needed.

5 Violence and anger

Promoting community mental health often includes dealing with violence, both violence happening now and historical violence. Whether experienced directly or indirectly, individually or as a community, violence not only causes physical harm but can cause fear, anxiety, and trauma as well as affect the social and political conditions that influence health, including housing, education, and work. This has led many community groups to make violence prevention and undoing the effects of violence central to their organizing for social change.

Anger is a strong emotion we all have. Anger can be triggered by violence or lead to violence. Anger can also be a response to social injustice and lead to social change. When anger is not channeled into an effective response, it can be expressed in ways that harm ourselves and other people. Learning how to pay attention to and transform anger (see page 85) can help all of us, especially children, to develop ways to understand, talk about, and respond to strong feelings without becoming violent. That ability is a central part of mental health and well-being, both for individuals and for communities.

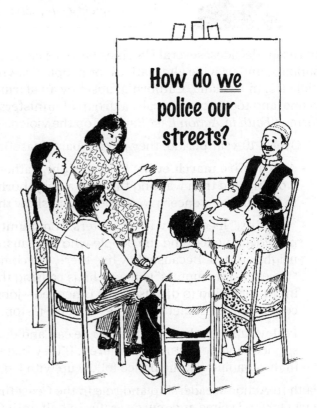

This chapter describes strategies developed by groups to deal with and respond to different kinds of violence and important examples of community efforts to address violence prevention.

Gun violence

The number of people who die in the US from gun violence is shocking. Guns are now the leading cause of death for people under 19 years old in the US. Countries with fewer guns and with rules that make guns harder to get suffer far less gun violence.

While the need for mental health support for everyone affected by gun violence keeps increasing, health workers and community organizers also focus on prevention—advocating to limit access to guns and to watch for and help people who might use a gun to harm themselves or others. Sometimes community healing processes—bringing people together around grief, rage, and frustration—are combined with prevention efforts.

Taking back the streets from gun violence

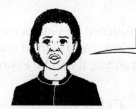

> There are more guns in the United States than cell phones! Our communities are flooded with cheap guns when they need to be flooded with quality jobs, services, and education.

In recent decades, several US cities have developed programs to identify, support, and provide alternatives for people drawn into violent crime and gun violence. In Oakland, California, upset by an alarming increase in gun murders, crime, and too many funerals, a group of ministers and community leaders formed *Faith in Action East Bay* to stop the violence.

Over a 10-year period, they put a 3-part Ceasefire Initiative into action:

- **A Ceasefire march every Friday night**, gathering at a different place of worship and then walking through a neighborhood experiencing violence to signal their concern to residents and show them they are not alone.

- **"Call-ins,"** meetings with ministers, community leaders, social service providers, police, and the people who are causing the violence in the neighborhood. Because they live there, the community leaders (called "violence interrupters") know who is causing the violence and "call them in" to a meeting to discuss what is needed—jobs, housing, drug treatment, counseling, or something else—to make it stop.

- **Follow-up** to make sure that people can and do take advantage of the services and opportunities offered. If they instead continue causing violence in the community, the police follow up with legal enforcement.

Faith In Action's leadership and role in the Ceasefire Initiative helped cut the East Oakland crime and murder rates in half until COVID stopped everything. Faith in Action East Bay has now restarted, confident in their efforts to reduce violence and promote uplift in their community.

Mass shootings

Although the number of people killed in mass shootings is only a tiny percentage of all deaths by gun violence in the US, their impact is enormous. A mass shooting is an attack on an entire community. When it targets a community of color, as they frequently do, it is a reminder of the racist violence that Native American, Black, Latinx, Asian, and other communities have endured for generations. It recalls past acts that were rarely acknowledged and almost never resulted in accountability or justice.

Following any type of gun violence, counseling for trauma (see page 34) is essential for survivors and the families of those murdered, as is organizing events that allow the broader community to grieve together. Ongoing programs and activities designed to strengthen and connect people within the community are a necessary and effective way to help repair and reset community mental health.

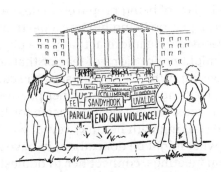

Temporary or permanent monuments and other public art honor the people lost to violence. These also provide a place to grieve and to renew community efforts to stop the loss of more lives.

Feed people, not violence

In May 2022, a white supremacist shot and killed 10 people at the Tops Market grocery store in a Black neighborhood in Buffalo, New York. In the aftermath of the mass shooting, residents pointed to how lack of investment in the Black community resulted in Tops being the only supermarket in the neighborhood. This structural violence (see page 79) helped sow the seeds for the mass shooting as the gunman chose the location precisely because it was the only supermarket in a Black neighborhood. Relatives and community members have taken many paths to honor those killed, specifically calling out the inequality and harm to the community caused by racism.

Community members have channeled their pain into activism by working to establish quality, affordable grocery stores to challenge "food apartheid" in Buffalo. Others give testimony in Congress, support efforts to limit gun access, and educate to highlight rather than erase African American history. People have also filed a lawsuit against the social media companies that fuel hate crimes and the online purchase of weapons.

Gender-based violence

Violence or threatening violence against someone because of their gender is called gender-based violence. Women and girls especially face a staggering amount of violence in the US and elsewhere. Violence is often used to enforce society's gender inequalities and rigid ideas about masculinity and femininity. This includes violence based on sexual orientation and gender identity—toward people who are lesbian, gay, bisexual, transgender, nonbinary, or gender-fluid. Forced marriage, human trafficking, and cases of missing and murdered women of color that go uninvestigated are other examples. Gender-based violence can be physical, social, emotional, or economic. No matter the form, it is deeply harmful to mental health.

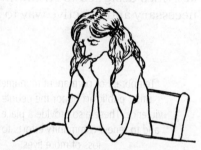

Most of us have either experienced or know someone who has experienced gender-based violence. Being aware of this reality and the different forms it takes is part of being prepared to deal with it. For example, a person being hurt by a partner might tell you directly or you might actually see physical marks. Or you might notice signs of fear or that something seems wrong. When a woman says she can't attend evening meetings, is it because her partner controls what she does? Or maybe it is unsafe for her to walk at night? Talking with her may reveal what is going on and what might be done about it: have another group member accompany her to and from meetings; connect her to domestic violence services and a place where she will be safe (both she and her partner will need help); or plan a neighborhood-based violence intervention such as a Take Back The Night march, where large numbers of people noisily walk the streets together to show how everyone should feel safe.

Sexual violence

Forced sex or any sex that is not wanted or agreed to is rape. Sexual violence also includes unwanted sexual touching, sexual harassment, and stalking. Sexual violence may come from strangers, but most often it is from someone a person knows: a family member, romantic partner, date, classmate, neighbor, or friend. Knowing and having trusted the person who assaulted you can make sexual violence even more difficult to talk about and recover from.

Many college students have never discussed sexual violence or do not know what to do if they witness or experience it. Non-profit *It's On Us* is building a student-led movement against sexual assault through chapters that carry out awareness and prevention trainings for peer-education. They provide students, especially young men, with tools to address the cultural norms at the root of sexual harm and instead foster a culture of violence prevention.

Support for sexual violence survivors

A person who has been raped or sexually assaulted needs first aid for any physical injuries. They may need medicine to prevent pregnancy or sexually transmitted infections. Most hospital emergency rooms have staff trained to support sexual violence victims and can document the injuries. This record will be necessary if the case is reported to the police, even if that decision is not made until much later.

The person needs emotional first aid at the same time. You can help them connect with organizations that provide counseling, find other survivors to talk with, and anything else they need.

Supporting survivors' healing process

The *Rape, Abuse & Incest National Network (RAINN)* is the nation's largest anti-sexual-violence organization. RAINN created the National Sexual Assault Hotline (1-800-656-HOPE) in partnership with more than 1,000 local sexual assault service providers across the US and runs programs to prevent sexual violence, help survivors, and ensure that perpetrators are brought to justice. Hotline staff recommend using specific phrases when talking to survivors.

"I believe you. It took a lot of courage to tell me about this." It can be very difficult for survivors to share their story. They may feel ashamed or worry they won't be believed. Leave "why" questions for later—your priority is to offer support. Do not assume that calmness means the event did not occur or harm them—everyone responds to trauma differently.

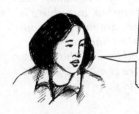

Knowing what to say when someone tells you about a sexual assault is not easy. Be as supportive and non-judgmental as you can. Support may mean helping them reach a hotline, get medical attention, or report the crime. To start, listen and let them know you care.

"It's not your fault. You didn't do anything to deserve this." Survivors may blame themselves, especially if they know the perpetrator. Remind them, more than once, that they are not to blame.

"You are not alone. I care about you and am here to help." Let the survivor know you are there for them and willing to listen. Make sure they know there are other survivors and counselors who can help them heal.

"I'm sorry this happened, it should not have happened to you." Acknowledge the experience has affected their life and the healing process will take time.

Intimate partner violence

The domestic violence prevention movement has raised awareness that violence takes many forms. In addition to hitting and other physical violence, advocates and activists also focus attention on harms from actions taken to intimidate and control others. Also, while most intimate partner violence is carried out by men harming women, abusive behavior can come from and be directed toward persons of any gender and sexuality, and happen in gay, straight, or other kinds of relationships.

Warning signs: Abusive behaviors are violence.
Control over another person can take many forms. Pay attention to signs of physical as well as emotional violence. You might notice someone mentions that their spouse doesn't like them to go out, or they worry about how their ex-partner treats their children. Other warning signs include a partner who is jealous, controls access to money and resources (like a car), pressures for sex or drug use, or threatens with words, actions, or both.

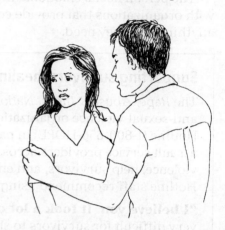

Understanding power and control

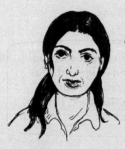

At the National Domestic Violence Hotline, we know that watching someone endure an abusive situation is difficult and it's not always clear how best to respond when you see warning signs of abuse. Your instinct may be to "save them" from the relationship, but abuse is never simple. Abuse takes many forms and there are many reasons why people stay in abusive situations. Understanding how power and control operate as a backdrop to abuse and how to shift power back to those affected by domestic violence are some of the most important ways to support survivors in your life.

ACTIVITY   Look at power and control in relationships

1. At the top of a large sheet of paper or whiteboard, write: "Signs of control and abuse."

2. Ask the group to list examples of how one person can abuse or control the other person in a relationship. These could be examples that are commonly understood to be abuse, such as hitting or always yelling at them. Add other ways a person is limited by a partner such as: controlling access to money, stopping someone from getting a job, not allowing visits with family or friends, constant insults, telling the person she imagines things, or limiting access to children. You could also group examples under categories like: economic, intimidation, isolation, technology, using the children, or others.

3. Talk about how warning signs often occur before there is physical violence and that some may be daily events. Discuss how it may be harder for someone to recognize these signs compared to signs of abuse that are more commonly thought of as violence. You may also want to discuss examples that reflect how family histories or cultural traditions consider or ignore abuse in how men treat women or how parents treat children.

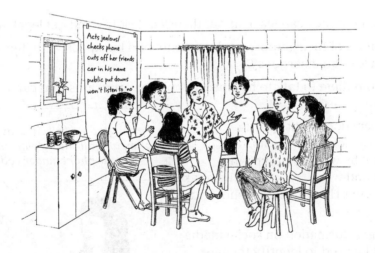

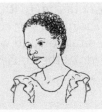

The Domestic Abuse Intervention Programs in Duluth, Minnesota, developed the Power and Control Wheel image used by many groups to explore these issues. An online Wheel Gallery (see page 165) links to versions in different languages and Wheels focusing on a religious or cultural identity, age group, and other specific situations.

Support for someone experiencing intimate partner violence

Be prepared to lend support by keeping a list of local hotlines, counseling programs, or shelters as well as state or national resources (like the National Domestic Violence hotline: 1-800-799-7233).

People who are experiencing or have experienced intimate partner violence need emotional and practical support.

Emotional support, as they process complex feelings and decide next steps, can include:

- acknowledging their situation is difficult and they are brave to take control of it.
- not judging their decisions, including if they leave and then return to an abusive partner.
- helping them create a safety plan.
- offering to go with them for moral support when they visit a service provider or legal setting.

Practical support, especially if the person depends financially on an abusive partner or otherwise lacks resources, can include:

- suggesting where they can get help with housing, food, health care, and other needs.
- advising where they can learn about their legal rights and get legal aid.
- storing copies of their important documents or a backpack with items they'll need in case of an emergency.
- encouraging them to talk to hotlines, people, or programs that can provide guidance.
- helping them document specific instances of violence, threats, or harassment by writing down what happened and when. Also help them take pictures of injuries and screenshot text messages.
- not posting information on social media that could be used to identify them or where they spend time.
- notifying (with their permission) specific neighbors or co-workers about the situation and what to do (and what not to do) if the abuser appears at their home or work.

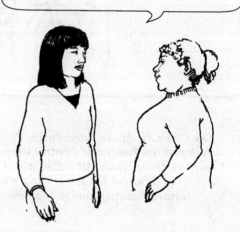

I'm so glad we talked, that you have a plan, and all the helpline numbers are in your phone under code names.

Help for the person causing abuse

In some cases, abusers may not appear to others as a threat, especially if they seem likeable or calm. The abuser may be good at presenting their violence as justified ("I was provoked") or apologizing and promising it won't happen again. People who abuse their partners usually need help to stop. Become familiar with local resources that help abusers to change. If it is safe, you can express concern and point out the harmful consequences of their abuse. Point out what is at stake based on what is important to them: they could be arrested, destroy their relationship, harm their children who witness violence, lose access to their children, incur legal or other expenses, or ruin their reputation. Assure them that with the right help and long-term support, a person who abuses can change.

Create accountability for those who hurt others. *Emerge Counseling and Education to Stop Domestic Violence* in Massachusetts has been working with perpetrators of violence for years. Their long-term, profound approach goes beyond anger management to help perpetrators address the root causes of abuse. Their Intimate Partner Abuse Education Programs center on how the person who commits abuse is entirely responsible for their abusive behavior and ways they can become accountable for their actions. They work directly with victim advocacy programs.

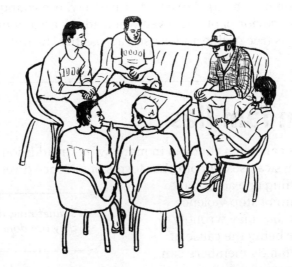

Healthy relationships help prevent violence

Most young people learn about sex and relationships from a mix of family and friends, school, music and movies, pornography, and social media. Modeling healthy relationships and opening discussions about communication in relationships, consent around sexual activity, and handling feelings are important ways to prevent sexual and intimate partner violence.

Healthy relationships and becoming an adult. *Coaching Boys Into Men* (CBIM) is a violence prevention program that uses the attraction of sports and the relationships between coaches and young male athletes to teach healthy relationship skills, especially that violence is not the same as strength. The program offers a set of activities built around brief weekly team discussions led by the coach. A single coach can do the program with a single sports team, or entire schools or school districts can get involved in promoting the development of a common language and understanding among young people. Discussion topics include identifying insulting language, disrespectful behavior (in person and online), consent with romantic partners, and talking through how the aggression promoted in sports should not carry over into relationships. In 2022, the program broadened its focus on young people's mental health needs.

Athletes are leaders in their community and other students look up to them. If they can model respect, non-violence, and integrity, it can spread like wildfire in a school.

The CBIM program has changed group culture to where young men now call out the offensive behavior of others, even when adults are not present. The CBIM curriculum is free online and is used across the US and, increasingly, in other countries.

Violence in families

Violence in the home can harm children in many ways. In addition to serious harm if they experience physical, sexual, or other forms of violence directly, children are harmed by watching one adult hurt another. Children cannot stop violence from happening, but they may wrongly blame themselves for being the cause of it. Violence between family members can leave a child feeling scared, confused, sad, anxious, or angry. These feelings can make focusing on school or getting along with others more difficult. Sometimes children respond to violence by acting out; other times, they become very quiet and withdrawn.

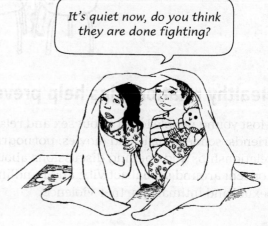

It's quiet now, do you think they are done fighting?

Experiencing or witnessing violence as a child can lead to adults imitating the situation they grew up with. This can create a cycle of violence that repeats generation to generation. Witnessing violence within the family may make a child believe that violence is a normal way to solve problems or show anger, and that even loved ones cannot be trusted.

Ending the cycle of violence by how we raise children

Children need to feel safe and loved. It is challenging to create a strong, loving family, especially for parents who were raised in an unstable or violent home or community (see "Structural violence," page 79). Encouraging open and honest conversations within the family can help everyone understand each other's feelings and concerns. Suggestions to help parents and caregivers end the cycle of violence and create a healthy environment at home include:

Be a positive role model by using respectful ways of communicating. Children learn by watching the adults around them. Show them how to handle problems and disagreements peacefully. When you're upset, slow down. Then use words to explain how you feel rather than yelling. This helps children learn to solve their own problems in a peaceful way.

Acknowledge your feelings. Use yourself as an example to show your child that it's OK to feel emotions, even when it may not be OK to act on them. Teach them simple ways to manage feelings, like finger-holding (see page 21) or focusing on breathing (see pages 31 and 140), and talk about different words to describe emotions, such as frustrated, left out, and worried (see page 85).

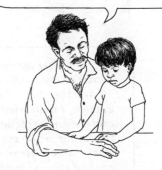

I shouldn't have yelled at you. That was a mistake. I was angry about my work day and that isn't your fault. I was wrong to yell.

With an upset or angry child, first acknowledge their feelings. If they speak harshly to a sibling, say: "I see you're unhappy and I'm sorry about that, but you know you can't speak to your brother like that." Remind your child that you understand how they're feeling to help soften the blow of any consequences or discipline.

Be fair about discipline. Clearly explain household rules, and what is expected of everyone and them in particular. If a child doesn't follow the rules, use "consequences" that are not overly severe and are related to the behavior, for example, taking away screen time if they misuse devices. That way the child will understand why their behavior is being corrected.

Recognize and praise good behavior. Parents and caregivers tend to focus on and criticize a child for what is not going well. Instead, regularly offer words of encouragement, small rewards, and special activities to provide positive feedback so children feel good about themselves and their relationships in the family and community.

Hope and healing from histories of trauma

Share family stories and cultural traditions to help teach children how to respect themselves and others. Southcentral Foundation is an Alaska Native-owned, non-profit health care organization. Their *Family Wellness Warriors Nu'iju Program* supports healing in communities whose cultures have been severely disrupted, as is true for many Alaska Native communities. One strategy is maintaining traditional practices through sharing stories on the radio and in person. This draws on community strengths to encourage storytelling as a way of teaching children, reminding adults: "Your resilience and your stories model how our words, our actions, our strengths have great impact on our little ones."

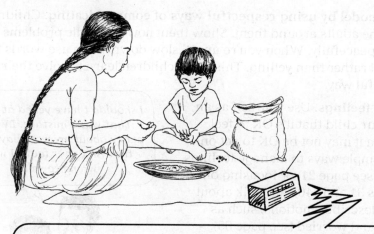

> I remember learning how to cut fish at the edge of the river as a child. I watched my aunties as they made their perfect and beautiful cuts on their fish and they helped me learn how to hold the traditional knife. Once I was old enough, I then tried to cut fish on my own. Though my cuts weren't perfect, and the knife frequently tore a hole through the skin of the fish, I remember the loving praise coming from my aunties: "You cut fish so good," "You are a fast learner." Hearing the gentle and loving words coming from my aunties inspired me and made me want to keep learning. Watching them and hearing their praise, I did learn, and today cutting fish is one of my favorite activities.

There are many ways to break the cycle of violence passed between generations. Some examples include Emerge Counseling and Education to Stop Domestic Violence (see page 75), the Milpa Collective (page 81), and the Occupational Mentor Certification Program (page 83). These programs are so effective because they respond to the particular histories and needs of their communities.

Structural violence:
Violence built in to our social systems

When physical harm, threats, and unfair limits on your choices or possibilities come from not a person but an economy, social system, or government, you are experiencing structural violence. The term structural violence describes how systems of racism, sexism, classism, and homophobia keep people down and affect each person's ability to enjoy life and have equal access to opportunity. By working to undo structural violence, we can prevent an enormous amount of lost potential, harm, injury, illness, and death.

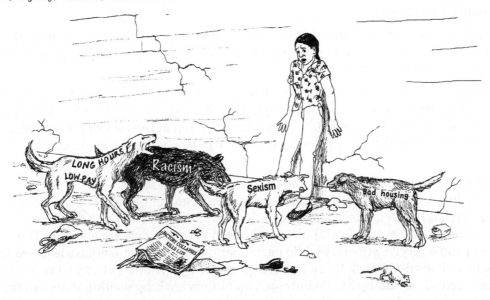

Structural violence plays out in society in interrelated and complex ways. As an example: We know that air pollution can cause asthma. Mapping where asthma occurs shows that it is highest in low-income neighborhoods, often where a majority of residents are people of color. That is where traffic, oil refineries, and other industries pollute the most. The schools get fewer resources, leading to a less adequate education for those children and, ultimately, lower-paying jobs. Racism and lower incomes often prevent people from moving into neighborhoods with cleaner air or better schools, and because banks historically denied loans to area residents (a practice called "redlining"), it is difficult to improve the houses and businesses in the neighborhood. This is the multi-faceted way structural violence works.

Structural violence can deprive whole classes of people of human rights: as immigrants fleeing violence who are denied asylum; Black men stopped by police who are humiliated, imprisoned, or killed because of racism; and all those denied health care or jobs because of their gender.

These examples have obvious mental health effects, but all structural violence harms mental health. Besides being impossible to escape, structural violence can feel both invisible and invincible because we are taught "it is just the way things are." Community projects that expose and combat these built-in sources of violence can be empowering, healing, and transformative.

Structural violence can lead to immediate tragedy, for instance, when a police officer shoots someone because of their race. The discrimination which is a feature of structural violence causes obvious harms and limits opportunities. One long-term effect of structural violence is stress that never lets up (see page 19). Persistent stress can build up and create mental health concerns such as depression and anxiety, and physical health conditions such as high blood pressure, digestive problems, insomnia, and others.

Medical research indicates that the effects of the stress caused by structural violence can pass between generations as physical and mental health vulnerabilities passed on to one's children.

Different strategies can help a person deal with the effects of structural violence. Counseling, other person-to-person support, and a variety of cultural practices can support health and well-being (see pages 22 to 24), but at the root of the problem are the harmful structures themselves, which can be changed only through social organizing.

Youth speaking out against lack of housing. Young adults at risk of losing their place to live or already living on the streets are victims of the structural violence of poverty and inadequate safety nets. A Richmond, California, organization, *Tiny Village Spirit*, works to empower unhoused youth and create housing. The young people receive stipends while participating in the organization's leadership structure. They develop skills and gain experience by speaking at city council and other meetings, by doing media outreach and interviews, by writing letters to the editor, op-eds, and social media postings, and by organizing and leading events. Youth set and meet personal as well as vocational goals, and focus on developing their life purpose and long-term goals. They move from being victims to becoming active proponents of why and how to transform harmful social structures.

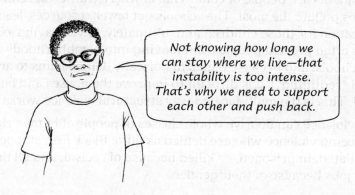

Not knowing how long we can stay where we live—that instability is too intense. That's why we need to support each other and push back.

Creating the conditions so kids grow up healthy and successful. The *MILPA Collective* is based in an agricultural region of California where many residents have Mexican as well as Indigenous roots. MILPA offers rites of passage programs and monthly discussion circles for youth, ages 13 to 25. Where children grow up interacting with gangs, violence, and incarcerated community members, the program provides a positive collective vision of the future, bringing young people together to focus on building self-confidence, resilience, and leadership while drawing on Indigenous and other culturally relevant living and healing practices.

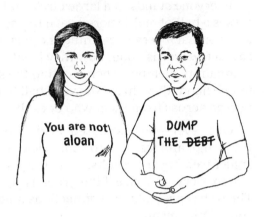

Stop debt from crushing people. The *Debt Collective* is a membership organization set up to be a union of debtors. They run campaigns to cancel debt (student, medical, bail, and others) owed to government and private companies. They also help individuals and groups to dispute and get out of debt. They envision a world where no one is forced into debt to survive.

Restorative justice to repair harm

Restorative Justice is a different way of looking at wrongdoing, crime, and punishment. Instead of declaring a person guilty and punishing them, the point is to look at the harms done to an individual or to a community and ask how those harms can be repaired. This can be done in schools, community settings, court systems, prisons, and elsewhere. While perhaps not appropriate in all cases, every situation addressed through a holistic approach, with mediated solutions that help both the person who caused harm as well as the victim, can help break the vicious cycle of violence in ways that simply focusing on punishment cannot.

Restorative Justice Partnership in Yolo County, California, has what it calls its "secret sauce" that creates connections through open and honest dialogue among offenders, community participants, and victims who choose to participate. To be eligible, the accused person must agree to take responsibility for their conduct. The accused person gives an account of the events that led up to the crime, allowing them to share the story from their perspective and provide context. Panelists then ask questions to understand the circumstances around the crime and work with the person to identify the harms that they, the community, and the victim or victims experienced as a result of the crime. At the end, all decide together the steps that are necessary to make things as right as possible, and to discuss how to avoid repeating the behavior in the future.

ACTIVITY   **Yarn ball web of relationships**

The *Yolo County Restorative Justice Partnership* uses this training activity with volunteers to demonstrate and get people talking about how violence harms community connectedness.

Everyone stands in a large circle and tosses a ball of multicolored yarn to one another. Each person catching the yarn ball says a few words about how they identify as a community member. Then, holding the string in one hand, they throw the yarn ball to a person across from them who does the same.

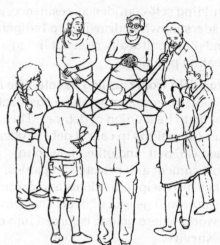

Once everyone has shared, held onto the string, and tossed it to someone else, a spider web of yarn results. (Toss the yarn ball to everyone twice if the group is small.) The web represents the connections among community members.

Then the facilitator cuts the yarn in one or two places to represent how crime breaks relationships between community members, weakening the entire web—the community as a whole. Tying 2 broken strands back together reverses the damage. By focusing on repairing the harms caused by violence and crime, restorative justice aims to strengthen the community at large.

Violence harms everyone it touches

People who are or have been victims of violence need support. So do people who have been violent toward others. Often, someone using violence has suffered violence and trauma themselves. Their experience may have shown them that violence works to control others or is a way to gain power in their life. Efforts toward restorative justice help people on all sides of a violent episode address their needs and strengthen the community. Though many places do not have restorative justice structures in place yet, you can learn from the experiences of existing programs and adapt their approaches to your context.

Understanding that those causing harm and violence may also have been victims, and that traditional forms of punishment don't tend to lower levels of violence, can open the door to approaches that interrupt the cycle of violence. Helpful approaches to situations where violence has occurred include:

Be self-aware and reserve judgment. Ideas about how to behave and the meaning of speech and actions vary from culture to culture, family to family, and person to person. What one person sees as angry or threatening may not match your experience. Open, respectful, non-judgmental questions can help uncover when differing cultural understandings are making a situation worse.

Be compassionate and aware. You may know or hear about a community member who has been violent with others or whose edgy, angry, or irritable behavior makes you worry they might become violent. Many of us are understandably uncomfortable interacting with potentially violent people, but it is important not to isolate them or leave them alone with their angry, irritable feelings. If you can involve them in community or other constructive activities where they can talk about their feelings and anger, and feel connected and understood, this will decrease the likelihood of violence. On the other hand, feeling judged, shunned, and distrusted can make violence more likely.

De-escalating situations that threaten to become violent is often a hard-won skill, developed through experience. By practicing to maintain a calm, confident, and sympathetic presence through your choice of words, tone of voice, and body language, you can learn to diffuse difficult situations. For ideas about how to prepare yourself and how to act in the moment, see page 62. Always remember to prioritize your own safety along with the safety of others.

Prison-based counselor training—offenders become mentors

Peer support among those who are or have been incarcerated is a good example of the unique advantage of talking to someone who "gets it" as compared to counselors who haven't lived a situation directly. Understanding the deep connections between addiction, trauma, violence, and incarceration led *Options Recovery Services* to develop California's first in-custody counselor training program. The Occupational Mentor Certification Program (OMCP) trains incarcerated people to understand the health aspects of addiction and work as alcohol and drug counselors. The extensive training requires participants to confront, tell the truth about, and deeply engage with their own struggles with addiction, past trauma, the violence they experienced, and the violence they inflicted on others. Upon graduating from OMCP, the Mentors work as group facilitators and provide guidance and support to other incarcerated people. Piloted in 2006, the program now runs trainings in 7 California prisons and OMCP counselors work in every prison in the state.

With their work experience and Alcohol and Drug Counselor certification, OMCP graduates often find employment with substance abuse and violence prevention programs when they are released from prison, applying their skills to carry on this work in the community.

Anger

Usually anger is hard *not* to notice. Anger's immediate physical effects can include changes in breathing, heart rate, and temperature. Like other stresses (see pages 19 to 20), constantly feeling anger can harm long-term physical and mental health. Too often, anger is expressed through violent behaviors, harming ourselves and others.

Anger can also provide positive motivation on a personal level, for example, to get out of a bad relationship or to find a better job. On a community level, anger can lead people to organize against gender discrimination or to improve their schools. Racism, exploitation, ecological collapse, political corruption, denial of health care—unfortunately, there is no lack of serious social problems to make us angry.

Having good mental health doesn't mean a person doesn't feel or express anger. It means they can understand what causes that anger and how to transform and channel that angry energy into effective action. We learn how to do that—successfully or less successfully—from our experience growing up in a family, attending school, and living in our communities and society at large. As adults, we often have to "unlearn" many of the habits we developed as children to deal with anger and try to replace them with more effective, less harmful ones.

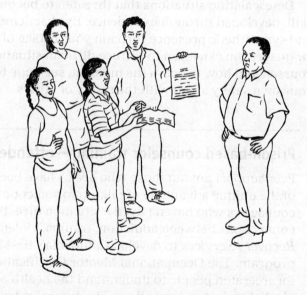

All cultures have various ways of expressing and acting upon emotions, including anger. Anger may be acceptable in some situations or when coming from people in certain family or community positions. In other situations, or from other people, getting mad may be totally unacceptable. But acceptable or not, anger is distinct from violence. While anger communicates feelings, violence is an attempt to cause emotional or physical harm.

The anger we feel inside, as well as anger and violence used on us, especially as children, can create mental health problems. It is important to develop the mental health skills that allow us to process our anger. It is just as important to change the social conditions that turn anger into violence in our communities.

Learning to recognize feelings and manage anger

Learning how to understand and process strong feelings as they appear is a valuable mental health skill for everyone. If children can begin to develop these emotional skills before they develop habits of violent response to strong feelings, it will help them, their families, future partners, and communities throughout their lives.

When children and young teens feel anger, they often lack the words to express what is going on inside them. It is difficult to identify where anger comes from and how to prevent it from taking over. Children (and most adults!) struggle to express strong feelings in ways that won't make them feel worse, harm others, or create new problems. Sometimes, when words don't work very well to express our emotions, art-based or physical activities can help us process them.

The activities below were designed for older children. Change them as needed to use with adults or younger children or to meet the needs of your group. Combine more than one activity to link awareness of emotions with exploring what works well to feel better or calmer when emotions become hard to deal with.

ACTIVITY   Working with emotions

Find new words

Build a list of words that help talk about strong feelings. The words can be those that kids already know, can come from book or movie characters, can pair with emojis, or can be part of vocabulary homework or spelling games. Include words like: disappointment, frustration, ignored, unheard, sad, embarrassed, ashamed, scared, worried, guilty, overwhelmed, hurt, furious, and others.

Make an "inside/outside" drawing

Ask everyone to draw a box with space around it or a person's head with space to write inside and around it. Label the top of the paper: "what you see." Inside the box, write: "the real me" or "what's really happening." The area outside is for writing words or drawing scenes that show anger: yelling, swearing, throwing things, hitting, insulting, crying, etc. Inside, write or draw feelings (see "Find new words" above). Use color markers to pair ideas, for example, if "scared" is the inside feeling behind the word "yelling," use the same color for both, or connect them with a line. Discuss how feeling hungry or tired can cause certain ways of acting, and add these words inside the box. Each person can explain what they thought while writing and drawing, and what they wish others knew or should do when "what you see" doesn't show "what's really happening" inside.

ACTIVITY   **Working with emotions** (continued)

Make a collage highlighting hopes and dreams

Using magazines, newspapers, or printouts of
online images, create a collage to show what
you are looking forward to in your life, want to
do within 3 years, or things you are grateful for.
Collage-making is fun and focuses on positive
goals. The collage can be taped to the wall to
remind you of good feelings and possibilities when
you are feeling down or worried.

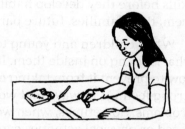

Reminder cards or poster with ways to feel better

Experiment with different ways to feel more calm or comforted when
distressed. Try squeeze balls, pressing your fingers together, pressing hands
on the knees, doodling, deep breathing, or other techniques. Practice several
of these as a group and then have each person draw pictures on cards of the
techniques they like best. The cards can be kept at a desk, by the bed, or pasted
onto a poster as a reminder of what to do when difficult feelings arise.

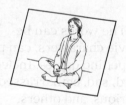
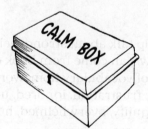

Shake it up and calm it down

This activity makes a glitter, sand, or "snow" globe you can shake and watch
settle. Making and using it helps you focus on how feelings get stirred up and
then calm down, useful for both children and adults to remember.
Have everyone talk about what stirs up and calms down their
emotions as you make the globes.

Fill a small glass jar or clear plastic bottle part-way with
water and a few drops of food coloring—choose a color you find
calming. Add a little sand or glitter and small objects like shells
or beads. For it to work well, add 2 drops of glycerin per 1 cup of
water, leaving a little room at the top. If you don't have glycerin,
use 2 teaspoons of vegetable oil or baby oil. Adding oil makes the glitter fall
slower. Glue the lid onto the jar. Shake it up and watch the contents settle.

6 Alcohol and drug addiction are mental health problems

Throughout human history, use of alcohol and other drugs has been a part of cultural and social practices. Widely available, they can be a routine and often positive part of many people's social relationships. But for some, drinking alcohol or using drugs causes serious problems. When someone becomes addicted to drugs or alcohol, it harms their physical and mental health and affects the well-being of those around them. And addiction can make other mental health problems worse.

Addiction to alcohol or drugs can be a lifelong challenge. Treatment can help people get beyond their addictions, though recovery is rarely "one and done"—a person may have ups and downs for a long time. For many people, alcohol and drug problems become like other chronic diseases where you can stay well but it requires lifestyle changes and perhaps medication.

There's no one solution for a person with an addiction and there isn't one path to find it. Harm reduction (see page 95) is an approach that helps some people where they are at right now, opening the door to other support or treatment further on. Most importantly, people dealing with addiction need community support for healing and finding alternative ways to have meaning and pleasure in their lives.

When does use become misuse?

Alcohol and drug addictions can be hard for us to recognize or speak about. We may fear criticism, blame, or shame because these responses are so common. It can be hard to know that we need help and hard to ask for it.

When alcohol and drugs cause problems in a person's life, usually it is related to how much is used, how often, and how much a person's life is affected by alcohol or drug use. Here are some questions that can help someone identify when their alcohol or drug use is interfering with their relationships and daily life, and becoming a problem:

- Is it hard for me to get through the day without having a drink or using drugs? Do I think about it all the time?
- Do I hide my use from others?
- Do I find I can't stop drinking or using once I start?
- Have friends, family, or a health worker shown concern about my drinking or drug use?

These signs are more serious:

- Has my alcohol or drug use made it hard for me to work, keep a job, pay bills, or carry out family or other expected responsibilities?

- Has my drinking or drug use ever caused injury to me or someone else?

- Have I ever done something unsafe or illegal to get alcohol or drugs?

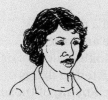

As a health worker, I ask these questions or have the person fill out a questionnaire privately before we talk. That way, I find out if this is on their mind and specific concerns without judging or pushing them. Then we can talk about their specific worries and what they might want to do about them.

Signs of addiction

Addiction is when a person is unable to control their alcohol or drug use, even though it is causing harm in their life. Signs of addiction that a person may feel or show include:

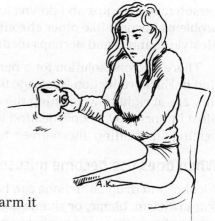

- physical problems when they stop using (called withdrawal), such as shaking, feeling irritable, or nausea; or more serious ones, such as mental confusion or seizures

- the need to use increasingly more of something to feel the same effect

- continued use of alcohol or drugs despite the harm it causes

Other activities that can become addictions

As with alcohol and drug use, other common activities can become a problem if they become too hard to stop or take over life in a way that is harmful. Most people handle video and computer games, shopping and collecting things, sex, eating, and even gambling in ways that remain healthy. But for some people, these activities become too much. Consider if you are hiding the behavior from others or if you can't stop thinking about it. Look at the questions that help people evaluate if their alcohol and drug use have become a problem (see pages 87 to 88). For example: Do you spend so much time playing video games that you have let

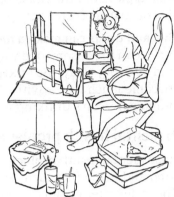

people down, ignore school, work, or family responsibilities, have new financial problems, no longer sleep well, or stopped caring for your health?

As with worries about alcohol or drug addictions, saying "yes" to such questions may show it is time to get help. If you are looking out for someone else, tell them you are worried about what you see them going through. It may help them to get together with others who have faced the same situation (see page 131). Support groups for these addictions exist for in-person meetings and online, and include 12-step programs (following the Alcoholics Anonymous model), such as Gamblers Anonymous (see page 155).

Addiction and mental health challenges can occur together

In addition to being a mental health condition for which a person needs support and treatment, problems with alcohol and drugs can make it difficult to tell if someone also is facing challenges with other aspects of their mental health. When a person is going through both, they are often connected. They can both be a result of the same life circumstances or hardships, one could have helped caused the other, or one makes having the other worse.

Mental health challenges can lead to alcohol or drug misuse. Feeling anxious, sad, numb, or having physical pain can lead to alcohol or drug use to get through the day. Using alcohol or drugs to self-treat current or past pain or trauma (see page 34) is also common. The causes of these problems can be difficult to identify and hard to solve, and people may try to avoid feelings and thoughts about them by drinking or using drugs.

Alcohol and drug use can cover up the mental health challenge or a mental illness.
Alcohol or drugs might make a person feel better for a short time by stopping their
emotional pain, but the cause of the pain remains. Meanwhile, their ongoing use of
alcohol or drugs creates new problems.

Alcohol and drugs can make a mental health condition worse. Feeling anxiety, for
example, can make someone want the good feeling that comes with drinking, but
instead of going away, the anxiety could get worse. A severe mental health condition
can become much worse with alcohol or drugs because both affect the brain,
changing a person's thinking and actions.

Both mental health problems and addiction need to be treated

Because mental health problems and using alcohol or drugs are so connected,
treating and managing them are also connected. For example: your friend is in
terrible grief after losing his spouse. His alcoholism has returned as he drinks to
cope with the loss. Any grief counseling would need to talk about the drinking, and
any addiction treatment would need to confront his grief and what has changed in
his life.

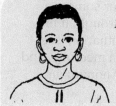

*In our program, sometimes people say: "If I wasn't depressed, I wouldn't
be addicted." But usually, that's not true. They will need help with
both problems. In addition to tackling the addiction, they will need
counseling and possibly medicines for the depression too.*

Talking about addiction

People with alcohol and drug addiction often feel shame about what they are going
through. They may downplay or cover up their alcohol or drug use, and avoid
admitting how it is affecting their lives and the lives of their friends and families.
Denial is often a part of this illness.

It may take a long time before a person with an addiction is ready to seek help.

If you think someone in your life is misusing alcohol or drugs, if they show signs
it is hurting them or the people around them, talking with them is a place to start.
If the person does not believe they have a problem, just hearing you say you are
worried may not convince them they need to make a change—but it is important to
try. It may be on their mind as well.

HOW TO   **Talk with someone about alcohol and drug misuse—are they ready to get help?**

The way to bring up alcohol or drug misuse can be similar to how to talk about other mental health challenges (see pages 26 to 27). Be mindful of your safety and how to get out of their way or out of the room in case the person gets angry.

- Don't wait until the person "hits bottom." Long before they are ready to ask for help, it may be on their mind or something they worry about.

- Plan to talk in a private, quiet place, when you both are sober.

- Start by saying you are concerned about their well-being and you care about them. Repeat this at the end.

- Mention specific examples of what you have seen that affects them, you, or others in negative ways.

- Do not judge, lecture, or even ask why they are using alcohol or drugs. Give them time to say whatever they want and listen carefully.

- Often people do not make any changes right away. They may need time to think about what you've said. But planting a first seed of the idea is something that may make a difference later.

- It is easy to feel frustrated if they deny there is a problem or become angry. These common responses are part of why getting help for problems from alcohol and drug use is so difficult.

- It can help to already know places where they can go to get help when they are ready.

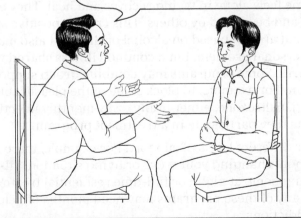

> Pooling our paychecks to cover mom's medical bills, I see you spend a lot on liquor instead of costs at home. And last week, I know you drove home after drinking too much. I'm really scared something bad could happen to you.

It can take many conversations before someone is ready to seek help

Because of shame and denial, it may take many conversations before someone with alcohol or drug addiction is ready to seek help. Besides family members, these conversations can also be started by friends, community health workers, and church or community leaders known and trusted by the person you want to help.

Family members need support too:

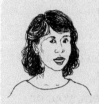

If someone is not ready to accept they want help, your life doesn't have to go on hold waiting for them. I tell the family members, "You have to take care of yourselves too!" Support groups can connect you to others going through the same situation. These include ACA (adult children of alcoholics) and Al-Anon groups. Goals are to focus on keeping yourself safe and emotionally OK and to avoid indirectly helping someone continue their addiction, for instance, by giving them money or covering up for them.

People struggling with addiction need support

As with other mental health challenges, shame and stigma block people from getting help to recover from problems with alcohol and drugs. When programs that support people struggling with addiction are made visible and available in the community, it lets everyone know where they can find help when they need it. Community education about addiction as a mental health problem—one that has social causes and can be treated—reduces stigma.

Treatment programs

Treatment programs offer the support needed to overcome addiction, usually by building community so no one feels alone in trying recover and heal. They are designed so people can help and be helped by others. This creates positive spaces and ways to be with others that are not based on alcohol or drugs. It also makes clear that addiction is not only a personal problem, but a common illness shared with—and overcome by—many others. Some programs may combine group support with medication-assisted treatment. For example, to block some of the pleasurable effects of alcohol and reduce craving, naltrexone, either orally or by monthly injection, works well for some people as they participate in a treatment program.

Treatment programs offer different levels of support. For example, there are regular group meetings without changing your work or living situation; all-day treatment programs, but going home at night; or full-time residential treatment programs. People attending any of these programs may need months of help and support to heal from their addictions.

It can sometimes take 6 to 8 months for the body and brain to make an initial recovery from drug use. When the effects of addiction have lessened, it will be easier to work on other challenges, for example, to figure out if a person is hearing voices because of drug use or a different mental health condition.

Meetings: There are many support groups that hold meetings that are easy to find and free to attend. Some people overcome addiction through religious groups, in part because they attract people who share a similar worldview and want the same changes in their lives. Alcoholics Anonymous is one of several 12-step programs that have helped many people get and stay sober. There are also programs that do not involve a spiritual orientation, such as SMART recovery (smartrecovery.org), LifeRing Secular Recovery (lifering.org), and Women for Sobriety (womenforsobriety.org). Peer-led evening meetings in local schools or churches can provide a space where people know they will be understood and won't be judged.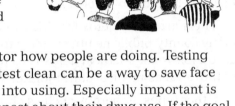

Testing: Many programs use drug tests to monitor how people are doing. Testing clean can be a motivating goal, and needing to test clean can be a way to save face with others who would otherwise pressure you into using. Especially important is that testing prevents someone from being dishonest about their drug use. If the goal of their treatment is to stay sober, testing can show how well they are doing or that they need different treatment or more help.

Residential programs: Although some people resist going into residential treatment because it removes them from their family and community life, it works for many people for exactly that reason: it is very difficult to change what you do when you are still living among friends, family, and a community that has not changed. Health insurance and Medicaid may cover much of the initial cost of addiction treatment programs.

The National Helpline 1-800-662-HELP (4357), run by SAMHSA, the government's Substance Abuse and Mental Health Services, provides referrals to local treatment facilities, different types of support groups, and community-based organizations. It is a confidential, free, 24-hour-a-day, 365-day-a-year service offered in English and Spanish. Also visit the online treatment locator: findtreatment.gov, or send your zip code via text message: 435748 (HELP4U) to find support near you.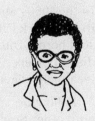

For people living on the streets, the combination of physical, social, and mental health stresses of being unhoused makes dealing with addiction almost impossible. We need more programs that provide mental health support and treatment for addiction while helping people transition into permanent housing.

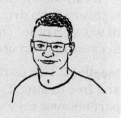

Our outreach includes talking to young people and others who lack stable housing. If someone wants to connect to treatment, we help with that. But we don't see their drug use as any worse than when college students or tech workers do the same. When someone's situation is shaped by poverty or difficult conditions, people judge them more harshly or treat them as less than human. That prejudice needs to be challenged.

Support for people needing to detox

When someone with an addiction stops using drugs or alcohol, at first they feel terrible. Their body reacts with anything from mild anxiety, hand tremors, sweating, and headaches to serious conditions like seizures. Someone experiencing withdrawal needs help to detox safely as their body gets used to the change.

There are many detox facilities, and community advocacy efforts have forced many county public health systems to establish adequately staffed detox facilities accessible to all. Medical detox uses medicines to manage getting through withdrawal as medical staff monitor you around the clock, often for 5 to 10 days.

Other types of therapy such as chiropractic care, massage, acupuncture, and various integrative and traditional medicine practices can help people manage withdrawal symptoms and cravings during detox. Massage, for example, relieves tension, which can help with stress and physical pain. The traditional Chinese medical technique of acupuncture places thin needles into certain places on the body to help balance body energy and blood flow, supporting both physical and emotional health. Good nutrition and drinking enough water are also essential during detox and through recovery to enable the body to heal and rebuild after addiction.

Community organizing brings detox acupuncture to the US

In the 1960s and 1970s, heroin addiction was a large and growing problem in New York City. While some people argued that US government agencies sent heroin into African American and Latinx communities to keep people disempowered, everyone recognized how the lack of effective addiction treatment services harmed Black and Brown communities.

Following a trip to China, members of the Black Panther Party joined with other South Bronx community groups to create the first acupuncture detox clinic at Lincoln Hospital in 1970. Acupuncture was combined with community outreach methods and social programs to promote access to addiction treatment, health care, and hope. While the government attacked and eventually closed the program, acupuncture as an effective drug treatment method spread throughout the US and continues today.

Community-based acupuncture and acupressure

Acupuncture and acupressure (putting pressure on key body points) helps people manage cravings and withdrawal symptoms. The *People's Organization of Community Acupuncture* (POCA) works to put acupuncture and acupressure "in the hands of the community." While certification requirements vary by state, POCA's Ear Circle program trains and supports non-acupuncturists to provide ear acupuncture. Called Auricular Acu-Technicians, they treat points on the outer ear with needles or with "ear seeds" (commercially available stickers that put pressure on ear acupressure points). These methods can help with addiction, recovery, trauma, pain, and stress. They can be used in mental health, treatment, and recovery programs, and in a variety of community settings. Training more people to do this therapy provides more than one kind of support. For example, when a POCA-certified therapist demonstrates treatment at a meeting, group members receive an important service as well as discover a valuable resource within their own community.

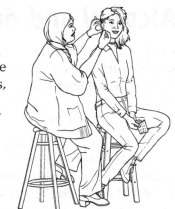

Harm reduction strategies

Strategies to make drug use less risky are called harm reduction. Even if people do not want to stop using or misusing drugs or alcohol, harm reduction can improve or save lives and limit harms by reducing overdoses and lessening the spread of infections, including HIV and hepatitis C. Harm reduction efforts include needle exchanges, ways to test the contents of people's drugs, and training on and access to naloxone (often known by the brand name *Narcan*), a medication to reverse overdose. Harm reduction programs can also provide a path for people to begin to remedy trauma, lack of social support, or other issues related to their addictions.

Another type of harm reduction for people with addiction to heroin or other opioids is to provide them with drugs such as methadone or buprenorphine (suboxone, bupe). They are much less dangerous, though they still create dependency. Medical oversight is needed to slowly lessen their use, and many people need them long-term. Methadone and buprenorphine are legal and prevent overdose, withdrawal symptoms, and cravings, allowing someone to work on other challenges and live their life without the health, social, legal, and financial problems that accompany heroin and opioid use. These treatments save lives and give people more stability.

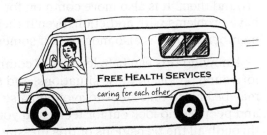

FREE HEALTH SERVICES
caring for each other

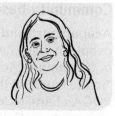

Our peer-run harm reduction program sees drug use as an understandable response to difficult life circumstances, and recovery as an open-ended path that leads to different destinations. For us, the most important thing is not whether or not someone is using, it's whether their life is improving and working better for them.

Alcohol and drugs surround us

Alcohol and many kinds of drugs are part of everyday life. Wine or beer is commonly served with meals, and both alcohol and drugs are often part of social events and celebrations. Advertising constantly tells us that using them is part of "the good life," and makes us the kind of people that others will like and want to be with. Ads never show people with alcoholism or dealing with the problems in the family it can cause.

Alcohol is often available in supermarkets and corner stores, and dispensaries and smoke shops make cannabis products increasingly easy to get. While the legalization of cannabis reduces the disproportionate imprisonment of people of color, it may lead to increased drug use in the community. This means our community organizations need to provide better education to youth about responsible drug use and drinking, make sure sober spaces and other ways to avoid drugs are available, and offer help and treatment when needed.

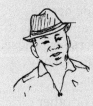

Guys pressure each other to drink in our community. We all live crowded together and there is nowhere to hide when someone says, "Just have one. It won't hurt you." But if a medicine you are taking means you can't have alcohol, they respect that. Also, if you say you are jurado, meaning you made a pledge in church not to drink for Lent or something, they respect that too. Our local priest hands out cards for anyone who pledges to the Virgin of Guadalupe. Then they can just show others their card.

Working with youth to prevent misuse of alcohol and drugs

Misuse of alcohol or drugs happens more often to people who grow up with misuse around them. It is also more common for people with parents or grandparents who have problems with addiction, even if they never lived with or knew those family members. There is also more risk if someone suffered trauma or abuse as a child.

Knowing this can help leaders of community programs or caretakers watch out for young people in these situations, and a person aware of their family history may be able to take steps to avoid misuse. In general, having community structures and people who look out for teens and young people, and providing caring support through all the transitions of this life-stage can help prevent general mental health challenges as well as specific problems of misuse of drugs (see pages 87 to 88).

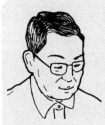

When kids use drugs, they are far more likely to develop lifelong problems because it affects their fast-developing brains more permanently. This is why programs that keep kids busy with sports, arts, and activities to help the community are so important—by delaying the use of alcohol or drugs for as many years as possible, it buys time for healthy brain development. Telling parents to "know where your children are" doesn't really help unless we are creating safe places where they want to go and spend time.

Spaces that are alcohol and drug-free

It is harder for people who have overcome alcohol or drug addiction to avoid using them when alcohol is made available everywhere and drugs may be easy to get. City, neighborhood, and community groups can design activities and events where no alcohol is served or where consuming alcohol isn't a central activity.

Our college campus has group housing run by cooperatives. Residents make, follow, and enforce the house rules. The largest coop residence hall is alcohol-free and drug-free. The students who live there can choose to use substances elsewhere, but everyone is committed to keeping substances out of where they live. For students who struggled with addictions before coming to college, this housing option is a life-saver.

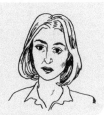

Turn down the money. The alcohol industry donates to community festivals and events across the US to associate their brands with generosity and to fill community spaces with their advertising. The North Dakota Department of Health encourages community groups to turn down sponsorship from alcohol companies and local bars so advertising and branded giveaways don't contribute to normalizing or making binge-drinking glamorous. Many events organized by tribes or held on American Indian reservations are also purposefully alcohol-free for the same reasons. In 1998, the city of Oakland, California, effectively banned all alcohol advertising by specifying that signs advertising alcohol cannot be put up within 1,000 feet of churches, schools, recreation centers, and childcare facilities.

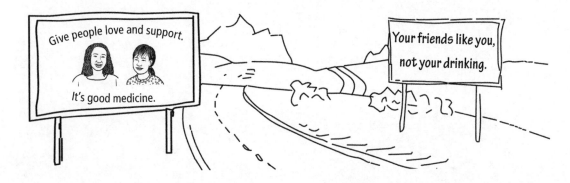

7 Mental health during different times of life

Some challenges to mental health arise during specific times in our lives, just as certain opportunities to promote wellness and mental health may be best taken advantage of at different ages. This chapter highlights promoting mental health during pregnancy, for babies and in early childhood, in adolescence, as adults, during aging, and when confronting death.

Babies come into our communities needing so much care. Creating healthy situations and settings for them—in families, neighborhoods, and environments—is central to their well-being and the well-being of our communities. So that is where this chapter begins.

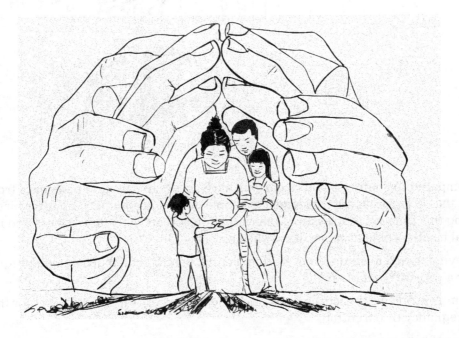

This mural from a farmworker community in Salinas, California, shows large hands embracing and shielding a family in the fields that provide work and food but also exposure to dangerous pesticides. *Hijos del Sol Arts Productions* with the support of *CHAMACOS* painted this beautiful reminder that the entire community can protect people during pregnancy and their babies from environmental harms.

Pregnancy and parenting newborns

Pregnancy, birth, and then caring for a newborn are big life events and people respond with a wide range of emotions to the many changes and challenges. Many people experience this as a positive though complicated time, finding pleasure, pride, and connectedness in becoming a parent. Along with all the joy and positive experiences, everyone needs extra support to get through the more difficult parts of pregnancy and parenting a newborn. After giving birth, a person may experience periods of sadness, exhaustion, and worry. Sometimes they may feel so different that they hardly recognize themselves.

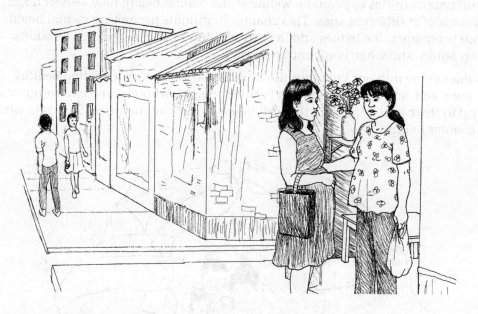

Compared to countries where parents have access to care and paid leave from work, the US lacks support systems for people during pregnancy and after birth, making this time extra stressful. Some situations create even more stress and make mental health problems more likely, such as:

- having mixed feelings about having a child, health challenges during pregnancy, or a very difficult birth

- family problems, including substance use, violence, or lack of support for the pregnancy or parenting

- lack of housing, income, food, or transportation

- lack of access to quality health care because of the high cost, racism, or other types of discrimination

- a baby who is very hard to care for, is born with health problems, or dies at or soon after birth

Ways to make it easier:

- Listen to how the person feels, what they are going through, and any concerns they may have (pages 26 to 27). Take care not to rush in with advice, especially if you haven't been asked to give it. Help people trust themselves and their abilities. Ask about and help them build on whatever strategies are already working for them.

- Make prenatal care and the birth experience as personalized, supportive, and culturally appropriate as possible. Midwives, doulas, and other birth workers may specialize in pregnancy, birth, or the time after birth. In some states, Medicaid will help cover the cost of hiring a doula.

- Organize friends or volunteers to help with meals, supplies, transportation, or childcare. Help for even a short time can reduce stress.

- Get new parents together to share feelings, problems, and ideas about solutions. Regular get-togethers help parents feel less alone, get practical support, and just laugh together.

- Arrange regular home visits and other ways to pay attention to parents struggling with anxiety, sadness, or a lack of energy that prevents them from asking for help or caring for their babies as best they can. In those situations, counseling, medication, or a combination of strategies may be needed to help a person find relief.

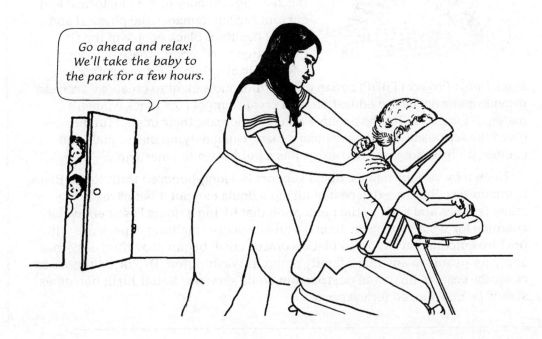

Better birth care

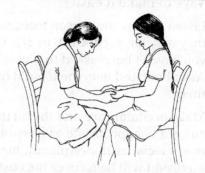

What if the process of bringing children into the world fully centered the health and well-being of the person giving birth? *Changing Woman Initiative* (CWI) is a Native American-led women's health collective in New Mexico addressing this need. Too many Native American women face bad birth experiences due to Western health care and bureaucracy. "We learned from our relatives' stories about feeling violated, unheard, and invisible to the world."

To meet the needs of Native American women, CWI offers home birth and other care in ways that validate and renew Native American birth practices. CWI's Corn Mother Easy Access Women's Health Clinic offers basic maternal and child health services while supporting mental health by affirming cultural identity. The clinic helps train Native American midwives and birth supporters and provides mother and baby with 6 weeks of personalized follow-up.

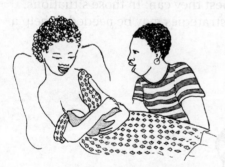

Black families experience more birthing complications and worse birth outcomes compared to other groups in the US. This holds true even for high-income families and regardless of the parents' education levels. It is glaring evidence of how historical and current racism damages the physical and mental health of Black people in the US. Committed to reversing these outcomes one family at a time, the non-profit *The Black Doula Project* (TBDP) began as an online movement to create awareness, provide maternal health education, and create support for Black women's maternal journeys. But the group wanted to increase their impact further given the seriousness of the problem: "Black women dying due to maternal complications is not just a sad story; it is a public health emergency."

Known by various names, doula support is a long-honored tradition in Black communities. But the extra cost of hiring a doula can put it out of reach for many families and adds to the perception that hiring a doula is somehow not common for women of color. To make an alternative birthing experience with positive outcomes available to Black women, TBDP began providing easy-to-apply-for grants to any Black family living in Washington, DC, or Baltimore to cover the costs of birth and postpartum doula services. Better birth outcomes should be guaranteed for everyone.

Depression

Many people feel depression and anxiety during pregnancy and after birth, and creating spaces to talk about it can help a lot.

The hormonal changes that happen during pregnancy directly affect your mood and the physical changes of pregnancy can make your body feel unfamiliar. These are some of the reasons why prenatal care is so important—talking about these changes with an experienced health worker gives you a better understanding of how your body and baby are developing and what to expect.

Lamaze (lamaze.org) and other childbirth classes, often provided at low cost or for free, allow a group of people to create community while building confidence about their pregnancies and giving birth. Classes like these can be especially helpful in communities where migration and social changes have disrupted the traditional ways in which knowledge and preparation for childbirth used to be passed down.

Depression is even more common after birth than it is during pregnancy. Because becoming a parent is supposed to be a joyous time, new mothers often feel ashamed about being depressed, thinking it shows they are unfit as parents or might harm their babies. Community workers can help families understand that depression after birth is common, ask how the person is feeling and what they think would be most helpful, and guide them to the support they need.

Depression can range from "baby blues" (mood swings in the first days after childbirth) to moderate or severe depression (see page 54). Any form of depression can be hard to get through but all can be treated with counseling, therapy that takes into account the needs of the baby, medication, or a combination of these.

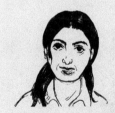

It's not always easy to tell the difference between common ups and downs and signs of depression or anxiety. Adjusting to life with a baby is overwhelming. New moms may think it's wrong to make a big deal about their feelings, or they have been taught not to complain. So we blame ourselves instead of seeing depression as a common maternity health problem. If you are worried about yourself or someone else, speak up. Good care can prevent depression from getting worse and can help you recover. Do not suffer in silence.

There are many reasons people with a new baby or young children can end up isolated. Limited options for jobs and housing can make it hard to live near friends and family. Politicians talk about self-reliance but often cover up the lack of government-supported community support systems. Because isolation makes depression worse, support groups for new parents can help. So can making it easy to participate with a baby in all kinds of community activities, either by offering childcare or making space for babies and small children to be part of your event.

Anxiety

Someone may experience anxiety for the first time during or after pregnancy, or if they had anxiety before, it may become worse. The emotional and financial stresses around childcare are big sources of anxiety. Local resources like parents' networks that compile and share information about childcare and other concerns of new parents can help a lot. Sharing babysitting with another family or a group of families forming a babysitting cooperative are other ways to take turns watching each others' children.

Make breastfeeding easier

Not everyone is able or wants to breastfeed, but for many, breastfeeding helps protect against anxiety and depression. So why doesn't society make it easier to have the time, support, and places to breastfeed? Why isn't paid family leave available to everyone? Some places even have laws that make breastfeeding harder! Activists involved with "lactivism" promote breastfeeding culture by challenging restrictions on public breastfeeding. "Nurse-in" events bring people together to breastfeed where someone has been shamed or hassled for breastfeeding, including in stores such as Whole Foods, Target, and Walmart.

In Pittsburgh, Pennsylvania, artist Jill Miller painted a colorful Milk Truck to create an eye-catching space for breastfeeding and drove it around to celebrate workplaces and businesses that support breastfeeding. Raising public awareness about the emotional and physical advantages of breastfeeding promotes mental health by undoing the stigma of shame and isolation.

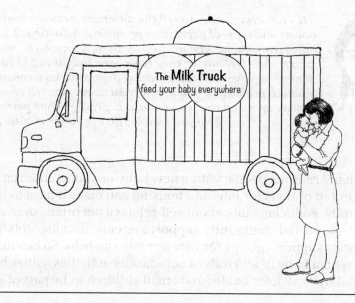

The **Milk Truck**
feed your baby everywhere

Trauma

Some people experience trauma during pregnancy, childbirth, or the weeks after. Trauma can be caused by a very difficult birth, loss of the baby, other medical difficulties or poor medical care, poverty or racism, or violence from a partner or family member. Also, given the intense emotions related to pregnancy, giving birth, and caring for a baby, a person's past trauma may be triggered.

People with traumatic responses (see page 34) during or after pregnancy need support. Help them get counseling, therapy that takes into account the needs of the child, medication, or a combination of these. Groups working to improve access to counseling and other services around pregnancy and birth can push the health system to recognize how much trauma there is in our communities and provide support.

Psychosis

People with psychosis experience a reality not shared by others (page 56). For example, someone may hear voices inside or outside their head that others do not hear, or see things that are not there.

A person may have experienced psychosis before or may experience it for the first time during pregnancy or early parenthood. Someone with a longstanding psychotic condition may be successfully treated with medication or another type of therapy that enables them to parent children successfully. They may need support and advocacy around their rights as parents, for example, the right to use medication to support their mental health during pregnancy even if the medicine poses a risk to the developing baby.

Psychosis that happens for the first time when a baby is born is rare. Postpartum psychosis is a serious condition that appears suddenly, usually 24 hours to 3 weeks after childbirth. The person may experience extreme mood swings, confusion, unexplained behavior, and insomnia, as well as see, hear, feel, and smell things that are not there. If their psychosis includes ideas about suicide or harming the baby or others, this is an emergency. Hospitalization may be needed to keep everyone safe.

Babies and young children

We don't often talk about the mental health of babies, but both their mental and physical health are shaped by the health of their birth parent and community, their caretakers, and everything in the environment they are born into.

We can support infant mental health by supporting their parents, families, and communities in welcoming and caring for a new baby. Making sure that families have sufficient food, shelter, safety, time together, and protection from the stresses of not having those things is very important.

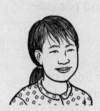

Why is there so much focus on children under 5? While learning happens throughout life, early learning lays the foundation for individual mental health. We learn most when the brain is developing most quickly—during the first 1,000 days of life, a child's brain is twice as active as that of an adult. That's why young children learn more than one language just by hearing them spoken. During this time, babies and very young children learn how to calm themselves, interact with others, and relate to the world in ways that will last their whole life.

Give babies what they need

As anyone who has tried parenting knows, it is almost impossible for one or two people to take care of a baby by themselves. In reality, it truly "takes a village." When parents do not get enough support, they can feel they are failures and blame themselves. On the other hand, getting good support improves the mental health and broadens the life possibilities for both the baby and the parents.

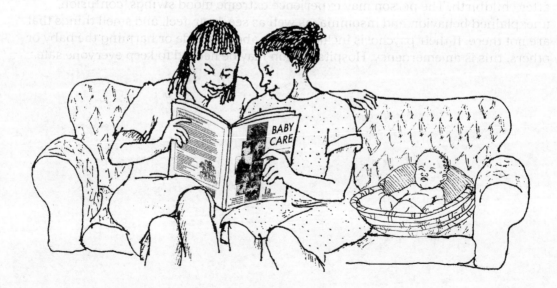

All babies need love, care, and attention to survive and thrive. Help parents have the time, energy, health, and emotional support they need to provide that to the baby. People, programs, and policies that help families with food preparation, finances, time off work, care for older children, and responding to health concerns all contribute to making the baby's world healthy.

- **Give parents** the time and energy to be with their baby. When parents get help with meals and looking after other children, the new baby gets more attention. When workplaces and laws guarantee paid time off for new parents—including partners and adoptive parents—time for bonding with a new baby is increased.

- **Give babies** focused attention. Newborns turn to the sound of familiar voices and respond to smiles and facial expressions. Each baby has different feeding, sleeping, and other habits. Spending time together lets babies teach their caregivers what works best for them.

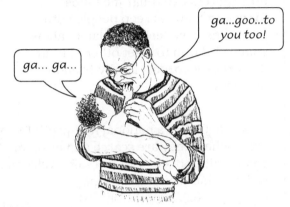

ga... ga...

ga...goo...to you too!

Sing or talk to a baby while you care for her. Respond to the baby's noises and talk about what you are doing. Babies like to copy sounds they hear.

Born to play. Play brings joy and comfort, builds relationships, and is a key part of learning. Watching a young child play and learn is watching growth happen. When they can safely explore the world and interact with others, play is a child's most accessible and powerful way to learn.

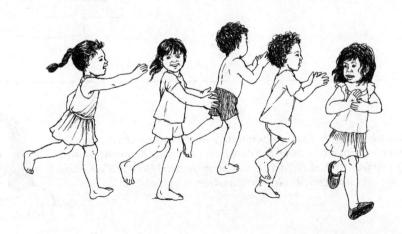

Smart spaces

Two moms created *Joyful Parenting SF* to make San Francisco, California, more kid-friendly. They urge restaurants and other businesses to add children's play areas and diaper-changing tables so parents can meet other parents. Regular meet-ups for young families keep people with newborns from feeling isolated, allow young children to meet other kids, and draw people to local family-friendly businesses.

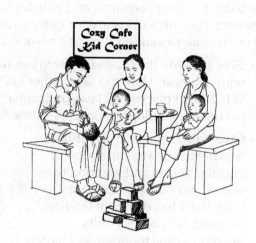

KABOOM! is a national non-profit focused on creating playspaces in areas where they are scarce and ensuring the playspaces allow families and communities of color to feel safe, welcome, included, and comfortable. Their website shares their *Playbook* (see page 162), a guide for institutions and community organizations to advocate for and create spaces like small play areas in laundromats and kid-friendly spaces in waiting areas where families seek social services.

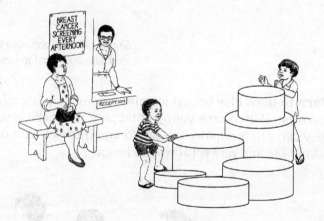

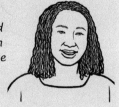

A question when planning any community meeting or activity should be: How will we make this work for new parents? Will the event be fun for young children? What childcare can be provided? How will we make it clear that their participation is valued?

Tune in to what children experience

Parents and other caretakers can learn to recognize and respond to their child's emotional state. This helps babies and young children manage their emotions. Without caring attention, children may find their feelings overwhelming and frightening, which can lead to behaviors that are distressing for themselves and others.

If you notice your child's behavior creating problems or your child is suddenly acting younger—such as having frequent accidents despite having previously learned how to use the toilet or no longer using words despite having previously been talking—talk to health workers or others experienced with child development to sort out how to help the child. Teachers who notice a child becoming withdrawn or not wanting to play can ask if the family has noticed changes too.

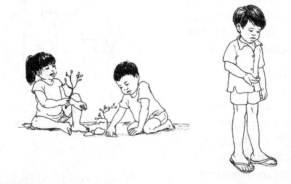

When a family is in a stressful situation and parents are unable to focus on or respond to what a child is experiencing, other adults can step forward to help. This can make a big difference in how the child will remember the experience afterwards.

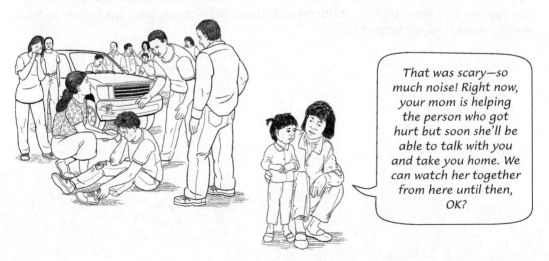

That was scary—so much noise! Right now, your mom is helping the person who got hurt but soon she'll be able to talk with you and take you home. We can watch her together from here until then, OK?

Separation

Separation from caregivers can be stressful but also promote growth for a young child.

Routine separations build confidence.

Though separating from a parent when a child goes to childcare might cause stress in the moment, the positive interactions with other children and adults will help the child learn that change can be fun and rewarding.

Unexpected separations cause distress.

When a parent goes away suddenly or for a longer period of time than usual, the separation can cause distress even if the child is well cared for and the parent returns safely. By maintaining routines and reassuring them that everything is OK, you help the child recover a sense of ease.

Traumatic separations require support.

Forcible separations, such as the death of a close family member, separation of immigrant children and parents, incarceration of a parent, and child welfare removal of children from their homes can be

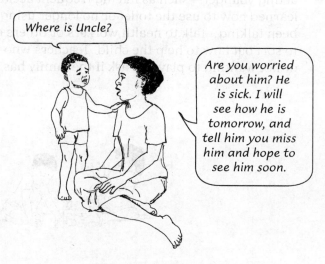

Where is Uncle?

Are you worried about him? He is sick. I will see how he is tomorrow, and tell him you miss him and hope to see him soon.

Reassure a child in a hopeful but honest way.

traumatic and have long-lasting harmful effects on babies and children. As a society, we urgently need effective ways to prevent traumatic separations and to provide support and healing for children who experience them. That support must include age-appropriate ways to help children talk about separation, loss, and other serious worries (for ideas see page 43).

HOW TO   Use puppets or dolls to help children communicate

If a child cannot talk directly about what he is feeling, he may be able to express it by drawing or play-acting. Because pretending can help children share feelings and ideas that are otherwise too difficult for them to communicate, "play" can sometimes be very serious. Use stuffed animals, dolls, or puppets to help a child learn about and express feelings.

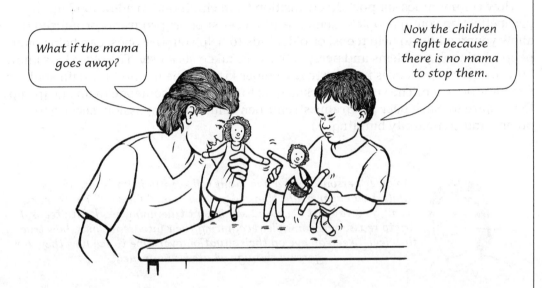

What if the mama goes away?

Now the children fight because there is no mama to stop them.

Puppets and drawings can help young children find words to describe and understand feelings. For example, ask the child to draw the face of a person who is sad, a person who is happy, a person who is angry, and a person who is afraid. Talk about these faces with the child. How do you know a person is happy? How does a sad person act? What does an angry person do? When do people have these feelings?

Make paper puppets with scissors, sticks, glue or tape, and pens or crayons. Or make puppets with scraps of cloth. Ask your child to name them and make up a story about them. Ask: What did they do then? How did they feel about it? Having learned more about what the child is feeling and experiencing, create a path through the strong feelings toward a resolution. For example, you can help the child wrap up the "story" in a way that leaves the characters calm or helping each other.

Adolescence

As children reach their teen years and begin to grow into adulthood, they experience dramatic changes—physically as the body matures, socially as they take on new roles and responsibilities, and emotionally as they explore who they are and want to become. Friends and peers are often as or more important to them than family members. They feel pressure to fit in and worry about being left out of social circles.

How communities support this transition from childhood to adulthood has a great effect on young people's mental health. Peer support programs organized to allow young adults to help teens, or older kids to help younger ones, can help young people feel their problems and perspectives are taken seriously. The older kids know how to share experiences in ways that younger kids can hear, and they gain skills as a mentor or coach. The younger person gets to learn from someone in an age group they aspire to. Such peer programs strengthen values of compassion, service to others, and community building.

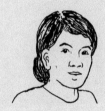

An older person knows a bad event will eventually fade into the past, while a teenager might think: "My life is ruined forever!" That feeling won't go away just because I say it isn't true. In my work with teens, I try to reassure them while recognizing their intense feelings, how true they feel. I keep an eye on their situation over time to see how they are getting through whatever happened.

The teenage brain is wired to take risks. As young people mature, they develop more ability to think through what could happen as a result of their actions. During puberty, with its hormone and body changes, romantic feelings and interest in sex intensify. Feelings that are difficult to control and a big mix of emotions can be a lot to handle and often lead to explosions of impatience, irritability, despair, or feeling distracted, nervous, or anxious. But learning to manage this mix of emotions leads to growth and maturity, and one of the rewards of working with young people is the chance to be inspired by their honesty, creativity, and enthusiasm.

At age 14, my son changed his name and gender identity the summer before starting high school. He was getting together with a mix of old and new friends and I asked, "Wait, do your middle school friends know about your gender and new name?" He came back a few minutes later saying, "They do now, I just texted them. It's all good." I admire how accepting kids can be—it is a good lesson for us adults.

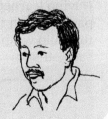

HOW TO   Work with young people

Show you know how to listen. This is true when talking with anyone (see "Being there for people," pages 25 to 27), but especially with young people. Listen without criticizing. Do not insist on giving advice. Focus on what they are experiencing and how it feels to them.

Help them flourish and maybe plant some seeds. Support them doing what they already enjoy (music, art, sports, caring for animals) and also help them discover new talents and interests. The same strategies adults can use—exercise, eating well, sleeping enough, building good relationships, and spending time outdoors (see pages 22 to 24)—help build mental health for youth. Keep an eye out for anyone who is shy, needs specific support to join in, or could benefit from other kinds of assistance.

Create spaces and places to connect. Community and school programs offering activities, sports, homework support, and volunteer or paid work opportunities provide young people with places to be and things to do. Spending time positively lessens the chance that they will spend too much time on social media or video games, or use alcohol or drugs at a young age. It can also buffer their struggles through emotional ups and downs.

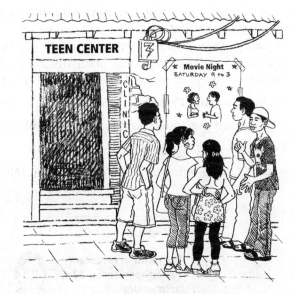

Recognize that young people experience "big picture" problems. Kids are very aware of the climate crisis, police violence, school shootings, restrictions on birth control, abortion, and other health care, and how people in the news fuel racism, discrimination, stigma, and hate. Like everyone, it makes them anxious and threatens their future. Support the creation of school environments, friendship circles, and groups that let young people challenge and change these conditions. Teens can gain emotional support, strength, and acceptance through participating in community efforts for change.

Life online

Most people in the US have a mobile phone by the time they are 14 years old. While internet access is now a necessity and social media may be interesting and useful, many apps and platforms addict us by design, making money for online companies at the cost of our mental health. We may not notice being sucked in, but then find ourselves thinking: "I know this isn't good for me, but I can't stop!"

Young people themselves are pushing back. Students have supported school-wide practices to store cell phones out of reach during school hours, except for emergencies. The non-profit *My Digital TAT2* helps young people navigate the complexity of being online and think critically about the benefits and drawbacks of their digital interactions, so they can make healthy choices. In addition to training students, parents, and health care professionals about digital well-being, they partner directly with young people.

In their internship program, high school youth meet with tech experts, learn research and presentation skills, and discuss the constantly-changing online world young people face. When these students do *My Digital TAT2's* "Digital Loop" activity (see pages 115 to 116), they think critically about their online behavior and share insights about ways to make it useful or limit it, such as:

- using "reminders" for homework due dates and important school or family events
- setting limits on video games or other addictive apps
- listening to music when feeling down
- when walking outside, following the rule, "No phone, instead look around!"

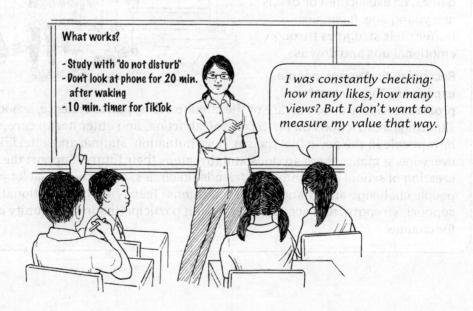

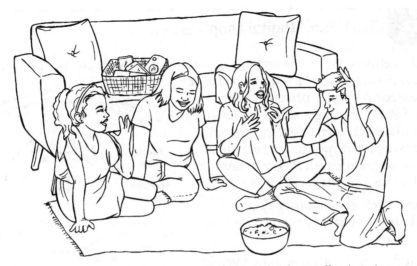

When we get together, for the first hour we agree to turn our phones off and put them away.
Then later we can take them out if we feel like it.

ACTIVITY   ## Chart your "Digital Loop"

Stuck to your phone? You are not alone!
Checking the same apps and platforms over
and over can trap you in a "digital loop." While
being online connects us to others and provides
useful information, it also creates problems.
Take a step offline to explore your digital habits.
Your family can do this activity, or a school
or youth group can use it to promote digital
literacy. Share it with your parents—they often
use devices as much or more than young people.

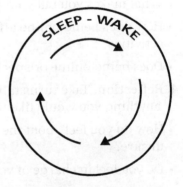

1. **Create Your Loop.** First, draw a circle. Second, around the edge, write
   the names of the social media, music apps, streaming platforms, and video
   games you use at specific times, such as "when I first wake up" and "when
   I'm on the bus." Third, in the middle, write the names of the apps you use all
   day, that are "always on." You can make your loop reflect a usual weekday,
   weekend day, yesterday, or some other example. Write down the hours you
   sleep and if you interrupt your sleep to use your phone.

ACTIVITY   **Chart your "Digital Loop"** *(continued)*

2. **Add Feelings.** Write the feelings you associate with each app. Does it make you feel: Connected? Excited? Relaxed? Stressed? Angry? Unhappy about yourself? You can also note the feelings that make you turn to an app: Bored? Checking for responses or reactions? As an automatic reflex? Try to tap into and name as many feelings as you can.

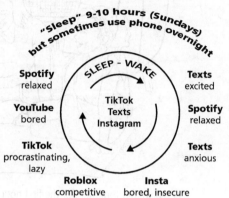

3. **Share.** Each person takes a turn explaining what they noted about their own app use.

- What do you check constantly? Which make you feel anxious, insecure, or take too much of your time?

- What apps or activities feel most helpful, happy, relaxing, or good in other ways?

- What feelings surprised you?

- What makes you put your phone down or get off your computer?

- How does being online affect your sleep, schoolwork, chores, or other activities?

- Does being online or specific apps cause conflicts with family or friends?

4. **Reflection.** Take turns talking about what you learned from each other and anything you would like to change.

- How do you feel about the time you spend both on and offline? Good, bad, unsure?

- Do you feel in charge of your time or is the loop in control sometimes?

- What changes (if any) would you make to your digital habits?

- Share ideas about how to balance online time with time offline to do other things you enjoy, like sports, getting together with friends, being in nature, making art, or others.

Variation: Start with step 2, with the group listing all the feelings people might associate with their phones and online time. Then keep the digital loop circle with you for the next day or few days. Every few hours use it to track what you do online and how you feel about it. Then use the reflection questions with the group the next time you get together.

Nutrition, eating patterns, and body image

Eating enough nutritious food is important for health and mental well-being, especially for teens. But instead of celebrating what our bodies do for us, our online time, mass media, and advertising often tell us there is something wrong with our shape and size, causing eating patterns that can harm our bodies and mental health. Too many people feel compelled to diet, binge eat, or purge after eating, or just dislike eating. Family, school, and community efforts can improve physical and mental health by changing how we interact with food.

Plan regular breaks for meals and snacks. Eating every 3 to 4 hours allows time to begin feeling hungry, but not so hungry you can't concentrate on anything else. Everyone can learn to listen to their body, be aware of their level of hunger, and see eating as one way they take care of themselves.

Prepare your own food as part of healthy eating. See what kinds of cooking or other food prep you enjoy. Learn which foods have what vitamins or what makes them nutritious. Avoid highly processed foods as much as possible and challenge yourself to try a variety of foods.

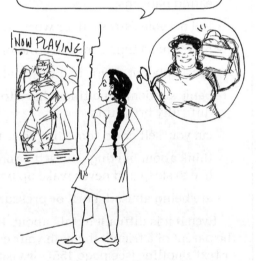

She looks strong and in charge! Just like my aunt who is the nicest, strongest person I know.

NOW PLAYING

Be aware of messages about body shape and size. Celebrating all kinds of body types and sizes builds self-esteem and is a buffer against social messages telling young people they look "wrong." Admire what people's bodies can do instead of what they look like. Avoid criticizing what or how much people eat, or how much they weigh.

I try not to call foods "good" or "bad," so my kids aren't always looking for what's "not allowed" at home.

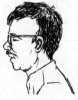

Try a "teen meal prep challenge," such as using a new ingredient or making a meal within a specific budget. Friends cooking together have more fun.

When young people need help

Adolescence is a time of vast change and transition, which can bring stress and anxiety. Learning how to get through it all is a big part of what is meant by "growing up." But when emotions overwhelm a young person's ability to function, when they express worry about themselves, or when they put themselves or others in danger, they need help. Share information about warning signs and encourage young people to reach out.

If you feel something, say something

If you feel stuck or overwhelmed, it's OK to ask someone you trust for help. Especially when you:

- can't fall asleep at night or have a hard time staying asleep.
- have very low energy or are not motivated to do things.
- do not want to eat, or eat a lot more than usual, or are worried about other eating patterns.
- feel nervous, stressed, or worried.
- have a hard time concentrating or cannot keep up with school work.
- use alcohol or drugs in a way that is causing you problems.
- panic suddenly and find it hard to calm down, with a pounding heart or difficulty breathing.
- cut yourself or do something else to injure your body.
- think about hurting yourself or ending your life, or feel like you would just like to sleep and never wake up because your life is not worth living.
- are being abused, hurt, or pressured to do dangerous or scary things.

Even if it is difficult to talk about, find someone you trust (at your school, the parent of a friend, through your church, a family member, counselor), call or text a hotline (see page 155), or visit the office of any health or community services you know about.

When you first talk to someone, you do not have to share everything about how you are feeling or exactly what you are experiencing. You might start by sharing just a little, enough so someone can understand the type of help you need.

Support parents and caregivers too

When a young person is showing warning signs or is in crisis, their family and friends are likely feeling worried and afraid. Just being there as a friend or neighbor can make a big difference. Listen to what they are experiencing and believe what they say about it. Offer to help out with meals, rides, or by looking after their other children.

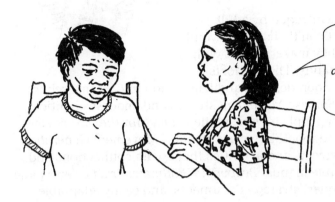

I know your daughter is having a tough time and you are worried about her. If you feel up to sharing, tell me how things are going for you this week.

Community support for young people

Many activities can lead to young people having better physical and mental health through building feelings of community, encouraging self-expression, and learning to make decisions and appreciate the results.

Coming together in nature. For nine years, the *New Roots Program* summer nature camp in Boise, Idaho, brought together teens from immigrant and refugee families for up to two weeks of daily outdoor experiences in the company of environmental professionals. The program worked to make Boise, which is more than 80% white, more welcoming to youth of color. Bringing together kids who might otherwise be isolated builds community among them, encourages exercise and new forms of recreation, promotes learning about the natural environment, and gives youth ideas about possible future careers. Across the border, *Nature Canada* promotes a similar program and created a toolkit to facilitate environmental non-profits to partner with diverse organizations serving youth.

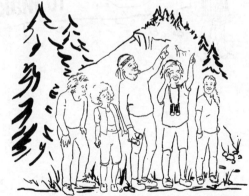

Providing a cultural grounding. The *Black Youth Healing Arts Center* in St. Paul, Minnesota, provides cultural, ancestral, and innovative healing processes to Black youth, including free classes on art, dance, and gardening practices of the African diaspora. Spaces and activities include a commercial kitchen, recording studio, ceramics, painting, weaving, performance stage, and art gallery.

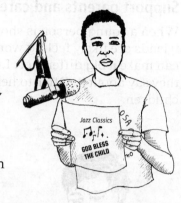

Supporting youth-led solutions. Outraged by adult inaction and the devastating effects on their future, youth movements are trying to force policy makers to act with the urgency the climate crisis demands. These efforts work to positively channel youth anger, despair, and frustration into sit-ins, school strikes, and demonstrations. The *Sunrise Movement* studies and endorses political candidates, and encourages young people to vote, while *Fridays for the Future* says: "Every day there are more of us and together we are strong." *Movement Generation* supports youth leaders through retreats and activities that create connections and mutual learning. Their downloadable manual *Propagate, Pollinate, Practice* (see page 166) includes curriculum tools, guides, strategy documents, and easily adaptable activities.

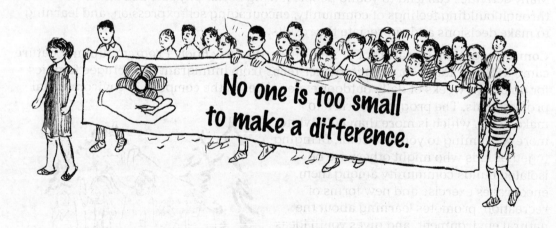

No one is too small to make a difference.

Turning trauma into youth leadership

Today's young adults of Flint, Michigan, a majority African American city, were among thousands of children exposed to lead in the public drinking water through decades of racist policies and purposeful neglect. The *Flint Youth Justice League, Flint Public Health Youth Academy,* and *Young, Gifted & Green* were part of the local response to address and help repair the harm, promoting environmental justice as young survivor organizers, scientists, and advocates.

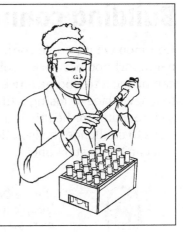

Inspiring hope with advice and by example. LGBTQ+ youth may face rejection from family or peers, as well as bullying or even violence in both public and private spaces. This makes depression and other mental health distress a serious risk. Individual and community programs are essential to supporting LGBTQ+ youth. *The Trevor Project* provides online guides and resources on gender identity, sexual orientation, and mental health and maintains a 24/7 crisis hotline (1-866-488-7386). The *It Gets Better Project* exists to uplift, empower, and connect lesbian, gay, bisexual, transgender, and queer youth around the globe. They share thousands of personal stories, post videos about many different personal journeys, and compile resources such as national call-in lines and local groups with supportive people to talk with. (See more examples on page 46.)

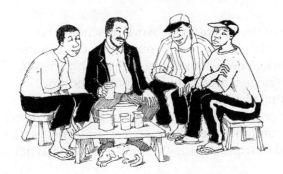

We can create "chosen families," people who may not be related but who do what good family members should do: provide unconditional love and mutual support.

Bridging the generation gap. *The Mother-Daughter Project* challenges the common negative stereotype that teenagers reject parents. The project helps communities form mother-daughter groups to support these relationships through the teen years, caring for the mental health of both by building trust and having fun in a group. Mothers (anyone in a caretaking and mothering role) meet separately for a few months before starting get-togethers that include their daughters. An important group rule is: "It's gotta be fun—or we won't come."

Building connections as an adult

Common ways people connect—through work, places of worship, children, sports, neighborhood networks, community service—do not always work for everyone. It can be hard to find new friends or a sense of community, for example, after moving to a new place or losing a life partner. Because personal and group relationships are so important for health and well-being, many community groups have found creative ways to challenge the isolation felt by too many adults. And if you can't find a group, you can try to start one!

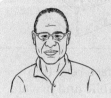

I have OK work connections but I live alone. A friend and I invited 4 people we knew to a monthly dinner with 3 simple rules: 1) 1 person picks up pizza and 1 person makes a salad; 2) if you host, don't clean before we come over; 3) if someone can't make it, the rest of us have dinner anyway. This has worked well for us for over 10 years! Sometimes we also watch a movie, but most of the time we just eat and talk.

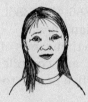

When I took on more caregiving for my parents—especially tough in a small rural town—I had no free time and triple the stress. A weekly 30-minute online get-together with 2 friends who are living through the exact same situation has been lifesaving. We can be totally honest with what is going on and I look forward to it every week.

"Third places." Many adults leave home in the morning for work or school and then return home again with nowhere else to go. Every community needs safe and appealing "third places" (not home or work) where people can gather with friends, run into people they know, or make new friends, preferably without spending much or any money. Cafes, parks, dog runs, playing fields, fitness and rec centers, libraries, senior centers, and community centers can meet this need if we put energy into making them feel attractive and welcoming. Often these are existing spaces that would be used more if there was renewed outreach or they were made easier to get to by providing transportation.

The Jarrell Community Library is not only the heart of its small Texas rural community, it is one of the only places to gather. Part of the broader *Libraries for Health Initiative*, the Jarrell Library has a certified peer support specialist at the library to talk to people and connect them to the resources they need. The Jarrell Library focuses on seniors, military members, and young families. Their mental wellness program presents guest speakers, stocks self-help guides and books on caring for those with mental health challenges, and lends kits that include jigsaw puzzles and other activities that help aging minds stay sharp.

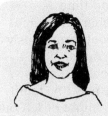

Our network of health educators helps others but we need to de-stress ourselves. All we needed was a space we could use once a week, a salsa music playlist, and a portable speaker to shake it all loose. It doesn't matter what you wear, how you look, or how you dance. I know dancing is good for my health too, but I go mainly because doing something alongside others feels great.

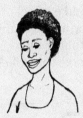

I have a friend who can't stay on top of her dishes, she loves to vacuum; I'm the exact opposite. When getting together to watch a movie, we first take 20 minutes to do these chores. Our house cleaning parties help too. Four of us meet once a month to all clean one home and rotate each time. More gets done, it's fun, and who doesn't feel better in a clean space? Sometimes our group will clean for neighbors who live with chronic pain or a disability, and they return the favor by helping out some other way. One guy helps us do our taxes!

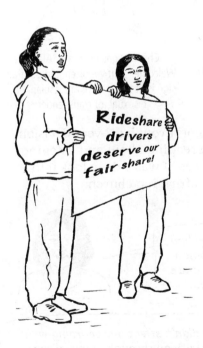

Workers working together. Many of us spend more time with our co-workers than we do with family members! Connecting with co-workers can make the workplace better (see pages 152 to 154) and work less tiresome. Maybe there are opportunities to take your break alongside someone else, chat over lunch, or commute together. If you have workplace improvement committees or a union, it can provide an infrastructure for social activities and lead to new friends.

Freelance work in the "gig economy" can leave workers more isolated and with fewer rights and lower pay than traditional jobs. Gig workers (for example, rideshare and delivery drivers, home-based call center workers) are coming together to share stories and strategies to improve their working conditions. In Mexico City, women food delivery workers connect via text in chat groups to share information and are supported by a network of cafés with orange signs in the window ("Puntos Naranja"). The sign shows the business will help workers in an emergency and provide a space to rest, charge a phone, or meet to talk about problems. These connections help build ties among isolated workers which can lead to improved conditions such as access to health care, accident insurance, and union representation.

Reach out to invite people in. It can be a challenge to break into long-time networks, especially for people who are shy, have just moved, don't share the same first language, or sense the door is closed to newcomers. When a group consciously throws the doors wide open, this helps meet new people halfway. To build community, go beyond opening the door—actively invite new people in! This shows, not just says, that there is space for them too. Noticing who might be new (the family that moved into the building, the student enrolling mid-year) or who might be left out (someone with limited mobility, resettling refugees or immigrants) is a first step.

Think about what makes your space welcoming and what might make it feel strange or unsafe. When you reach out, are you aware of people's languages, family obligations, access to transport, and other constraints (see page 10) that could limit participation? Ask about and respond to what people need to make them feel welcomed into your circle.

New faces bring new learning

Since 1972, LGBTQ+ members of the United Church of Christ (UCC) created an *Open and Affirming Coalition* to raise consciousness about how LGBTQ+ individuals and their families need and deserve to feel welcome and safe in their churches, and now hundreds of UCC-affiliated churches have worked toward that goal.

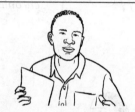

Church signs may say: "All Are Welcome." But we often find out that sign isn't for us if we are lesbian, gay, bisexual, or transgender.

The UCC Longmeadow, Massachusetts, church went through a 2-year decision-making process that included Bible reflection and reading about and listening to LGBTQ+ identified people's first-hand experiences. It was a deep look into what it really meant to "come out" as an open and affirming church.

When my fellow church members learned about my bad experience in another church as a transgender woman, they took on the work to create a truly welcoming space.

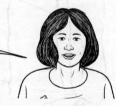

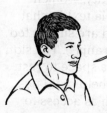

I used to think homophobia didn't affect me. Learning what people in the LGBTQ+ community go through in mixed spaces like ours and how to be an ally was transformative for me. I am deeply proud of our church's open and affirming practices and glad to see our church grow as a result. And I feel really blessed with all the new friendships I have made.

Aging and living as an older person

As people get older, many of their avenues of social interaction narrow or disappear, leading to more loneliness, anxiety, and depression. Depression and anxiety are made worse by weak goverment support for people who are aging. Social Security income, when people qualify for it, rarely provides enough to live on, and the increasing privatization and costs of Medicare make health care more complicated and harder to get. Many communities lack services for people as they get older.

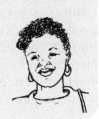

It isn't right that life is so hard for older people. There should be more help available and it should be easier to get. To find public and non-profit programs and other resources that may be near you (grouped as Area Agencies on Aging), look at: eldercare.acl.gov. *These federal, state, and local programs might offer daytime care, caregiver training, respite care, and help for people applying to programs like Medicare and Medicaid.*

The close relationship between physical and mental health (see page 20) makes combining many activities in places like senior centers a great way to strengthen elders individually and as a community. By providing nutritious lunches, dance classes and chair yoga, card games, and book and movie discussions, older people take advantage of opportunities to socialize and fight isolation while their families and caregivers get a break.

Multi-generational solutions. Matching older people seeking companionship and household help with younger people who need housing and enjoy helping creates a win-win situation. In fact, any kind of connecting across generations often improves everyone's mental health while addressing basic needs.

The *Southeast Arizona Health Education Center* (SEAHEC) works to improve health and well-being in US rural border and migrant communities. SEAHEC's *Entre Nosotros* curriculum trains community health workers to support elders to look out for each other's mental health and recognize warning signs, learn overdose prevention, and learn techniques that help people feel calm. SEAHEC's Future/Youth Health Leaders Club prompted high school students to interview people in group care homes about their interests and needs. They designed and hung posters in Spanish and English to brighten rooms and moods, organized intergenerational Bingo and *Lotería* games, distributed holiday gift baskets, and made lasting friendships.

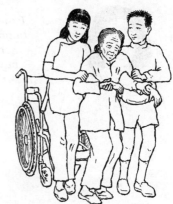

Peer helpers. *The Village to Village Network* helps groups set up support networks among elders to meet different needs (like transportation, technology assistance, home repair, and errands). They also sponsor activities and outings. They help keep people healthy, connected, and more independent.

Transportation. Many seniors can no longer drive or walk distances, and need support getting to and from the grocery store, doctor's appointments, the library, and other places. City-sponsored on-call senior shuttles or free ride vouchers can provide needed and dependable transportation.

Listening ears. A volunteer at a suicide prevention hotline in San Francisco, California, noticed that many older callers were not talking about suicide, but were lonely and looking for somebody to talk with. He started a *Friendship Line* (now in English and Spanish) to provide a "listening ear" for callers. It also offers telephone medication reminders, well-being checks, and even in-person visits. If there is not a local call-in line near you, try the national *Friendly Voice* line and speak to an AARP-trained volunteer. For call-in lines and hotline numbers, see page 155.

Document community history. Organize, train, and support young people to interview long-time neighborhood residents and record their memories of the community and what has changed. Compiling and sharing oral histories builds community pride, honors the life experiences of elders, and validates the creative work of young documentarians.

Protect against elder abuse and scams. Promote conversations among family members to help people plan for a time when they will not be able to look after their own finances. Getting the word out about how to recognize and deal with common scams helps protect seniors and begins to address the shame and grief resulting when someone is tricked into giving away money. The *AARP Fraud Watch Network and Volunteers of America* created the VOA | ReST program (Resilience, Strength, and Time) to help people through the emotional impact of these experiences, offering facilitated peer discussion groups.

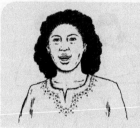

I knew my mom would be upset if I said, "I need access to your finances in case your memory loss gets worse." Instead, I asked her to tell me more about my aunt who spent all her money buying items online she already had. Then I said, "I want to make sure that never happens to you." That opened the door for us to make a plan.

Alliances to change the care economy and the nature of care work. Eldercare Dialogues grew out of activism by the *National Domestic Workers' Alliance* and brought together elders, direct care workers, and family members in conversations. With a focus on transforming care jobs into "good jobs," with adequate pay and decent conditions, they developed policy recommendations, standards for being a good employer, and a training guide for anyone to start similar conversations (see page 166). *Caring Across Generations* is a national organization also focused on the dignity deserved by both caregivers and those needing care. They record stories and create public awareness campaigns to transform attitudes and narratives about aging, disability, and care. They also lobby for policy changes at every level.

Death and dying

Thinking ahead to and preparing for death can bring up strong emotions. Dying and death are topics people often avoid talking about, even among friends and family. For many, not being able to talk about and plan for death creates stress, anxiety, and depression.

Let's talk about it. "Death Cafes" are one-time or multi-part group conversations to talk about death in an open, respectful, supportive, and confidential space so people can feel safe expressing their thoughts. Talking freely about death can remove the taboo against talking about it, provide relief for participants, and lead to sharing new ways to think about the end of life. With tips on how to keep it simple, the *Death Cafe Guide* (free from deathcafe.com) covers how to organize an event, often in a library or other public space, and how to make everyone who attends feel welcome.

Make your wishes known. It should be easier to think about and get legal support for what you want for your end of life, including in case of an emergency. Some libraries and legal aid non-profits hold clinics to help write an Advance Health Care Directive, a document that specifies the medical care you want under certain conditions (for example, not wanting machines to keep your heart pumping if you have brain damage and won't wake up). Legal aid clinics can also help you write a simple Last Will and Testament. Making these decisions when you are well, and adjusting them as needed, can bring you and your family peace of mind. *PREPARE for your care* (prepareforyourcare.org) walks you through this process based on the state you live in.

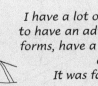

I have a lot of single friends, working in different professions who want to have an advance health directive but put it off. We decided to get the forms, have a party to fill out and print them, and then be witnesses for each other, signing them to make them legal.
It was fast and fun—and we felt good about getting it done!

Prepare and share a list of palliative care, complementary care, and hospice services. Help people learn about these services, how to access them, and which are free or affordable. *Palliative care* focuses on well-being, comfort, and support to make decisions so a person will feel better. It is not only for people who are dying. *Complementary care* means therapies that help ease problems from illness, lessen treatment's side effects, and feel calmer and worry less, such as meditation, herbal remedies, pain medicines, special diets, exercise, hypnosis, acupuncture, massage, and prayer or spiritual healing. *Hospice services* focus on making a person who is dying more comfortable by reducing pain and other symptoms with medication and other methods, helping them and their family make plans, find emotional and spiritual support, and address other needs. Hospice can start months before the end of life and can happen in a hospice center, a hospital, or where a person lives.

Spending time with someone who is dying

When you are with someone who is dying, it can be hard to know what to say. Still, many people find this time to be meaningful and important. It can provide a chance to give both the person and yourself peace of mind. If there are important things that remain unsaid between you, you will need to decide how you want to express your thoughts and feelings.

It may feel right to simply be present, perhaps holding the person's hand so they know you are there for them. Regardless of whether they have months to live or are no longer fully conscious, you can:

- talk about memories, especially happy ones, and accomplishments the person can feel good about.
- thank the person for what they have given you.
- let the person know you love them and will miss them.
- express forgiveness or ask for forgiveness.

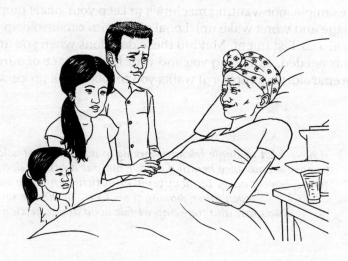

Sometimes, confronting the end of life may find you or the dying person angry, sad, or scared. Staying close, keeping them company, and listening can show you care. You do not have to express feelings that you do not have or tell them what they want to hear. You will have to live with your last interactions with them after they pass away. If what you feel you must say may be difficult for them to hear, try to say it in a way you will not later regret.

Sometimes a person wants to talk about dying and may ask you what it will be like. It can be hard to hear these questions when there are no easy answers. It is OK to say: "I don't know. Nobody does." You can reassure the person that medications and other methods are available to help control pain.

Every person's body slows differently as they die. Holding their hand as they cry or talk about their good memories or regrets may be the best you can do. Telling them you will be there with them as they die can help, even after they lose the ability to speak. They may appreciate prayers, other religious or spiritual practices, music, or incense. Often the person can still hear you even when they no longer seem to be awake or responding. Just sitting with someone and breathing with them can be very comforting in the last stages of dying. Saying out loud that it is OK for the person to let go can make a difference. They may need pain medication along with your care and presence to bring comfort and ease their transition to death.

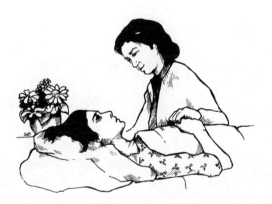

A dying person and their family need care with love and dignity. With death as a part of life, hospice workers, death doulas, and health promoters trained in what is needed at the end of life accompany families and share their skills to help people get through the hardest of times.

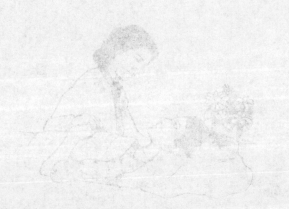

8 Support groups

Meeting with others who share a similar experience can be a source of support. This is especially true for situations that are hard or uncomfortable to talk about.

Being with others rather than being alone can bring some comfort. Hearing others speak about their experiences can help you think about your own. For example, when parents who know the grief of losing a child lead a support group, sharing the hard experience they have gained can help other participants feel less alone and overwhelmed.

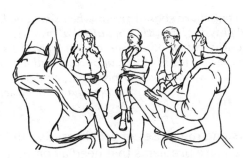

A group can also address specific problems together. This increases the possibility of creating change and increases the benefits of the healing companionship of working with others.

Support groups help in many ways

Recognize feelings. People often hide their feelings or do not even recognize they have them because they think their feelings are bad, shameful, or a sign of weakness, or because in their family or culture, people tend to hide or ignore feelings rather than talk about them. Hearing others talk about feelings can help people recognize and think about their own.

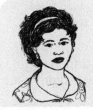

Before, I blamed myself for my husband's anger issues and problems with alcohol. I thought: Why would I want to talk with anyone about my failures? But my neighbor brought me to her group where everyone had a partner who drank too much. I began to realize it was not my fault, and making excuses for my husband was not helpful for either of us.

Know you aren't alone. Sharing with and listening to other people, in person or online, often shows that others have faced similar situations, provides relief and comfort, and can give you ideas about what to do next.

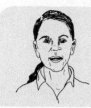

We all had grown up witnessing abuse and alcoholism but we had never talked about it with others or worked through how it affected us. It was a huge relief to share our stories.

Get support. Feeling bad can make you feel drained and discouraged. Meeting as a group gives people energy and ideas, helping everyone cope with their daily problems. Group members can also check in with each other between meetings.

In our church-based group, when someone has a rough day, one of us will pray for her with a beautiful affirmation, describing out loud all the positive things about her, calling forth the strength she needs to heal. The person feels totally supported, and listening gives us all focus. Even though we all have our problems, channeling our collective love makes bearing them easier.

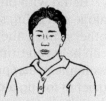

Understand the causes of problems. By talking together, we come to realize that many people share problems that need a common solution. This helps identify root causes in society and stops us from just blaming ourselves.

Identify solutions. Groups can come up with possible solutions to problems, evaluate them, and decide what to do. They can also help us think about the obstacles that might get in the way of a solution and how to overcome these.

I was ready to come out to my family about my sexuality but was worried about how it would go. Hearing how others in our group kept their family relations intact was a relief and helped me see what I could try with my family.

Recognize strengths. The group can ask: "What are you most proud of?" and "What do you think you handled well?" As people get to know each other, they will also be able to remind each person of all their strengths and skills and how they have handled distressing feelings and overcome challenges before.

Build power together. Acting together is always more powerful than acting alone. When a group identifies a community problem to improve, knowing that some or all of you can work on it together makes fixing it seem more possible.

Celebrate, commemorate, and have fun. Build community by celebrating birthdays or other occasions, and do other activities besides talking. Change things up! Bring in someone to lead a healing technique, or have members take turns organizing games and energizing activities. A group focused on personal goals, for example, staying sober, might mark reaching a milestone with a song, food, or a simple gift.

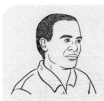

Sometimes people are sent to a group without it being their idea. Others try out a group and decide it's not for them. It can be the right decision when someone chooses to leave a group when it isn't a good fit. Groups work best when people want to be there.

Starting a support group

Anyone can start a support group. It just takes a few people who can meet regularly and have something in common. People may get together because they share the same challenges or have similar experiences, or because they live in the same neighborhood, have children at the same school, worship at the same church, or work at the same job. Sometimes a health worker or teacher will start and participate in a group, but often professionals are only involved when they are invited to attend a meeting as a resource person. A group needs to discuss and agree upon:

When and where to meet. It helps to have a quiet place with enough privacy to make people feel comfortable talking, perhaps a space in a community center, library, school, or place of worship. Choose a meeting day and time that allows the most people to participate. Make sure the space is accessible for someone with mobility issues, and see if providing childcare or anything else will make it easier for more people to join. If the group meets online, or mixes being in-person with being online, see if tech advice or access to digital devices is needed. Get help getting online from human-i-t.org or pcsforpeople.org.

What you hope to do. Have the group choose the topics to talk about. Give everyone a chance to express what they would like from the group: to talk about feelings, to share ideas about facing certain situations, to learn healing techniques, or something else. Try to keep expectations realistic. Support groups can be helpful in many ways, but they will not fix everything. (See pages 143 to 145 for ideas about handling the stresses that may arise in support groups.)

Share ideas about preferred words. Talk about any specific words that people would prefer to use or not use, so everyone is aware of these concerns. Even if there are differences in opinion about how people understand and use certain words, the group can commit to respect how each member wants to talk about themselves.

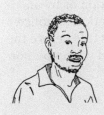

In our group, even though everyone had gotten a diagnosis saying they were "mentally ill," some preferred saying they had survived trauma, had a spiritual emergency, had mental distress, or had other ways to refer to it. We talked a lot about how some terms ignore or erase who people are. We agreed each person could use the words that worked for them and that group members would work to respect that.

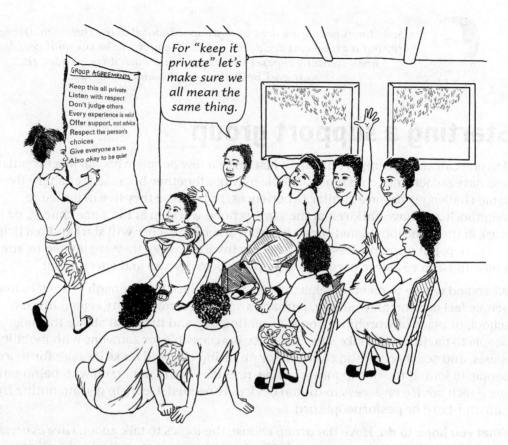

Group agreements. While agreements can be added or changed as you go along, it is good to begin by deciding on basic rules so everyone feels safe about participating and sharing. One basic agreement might be to keep group discussions private. Another might be to avoid judging people or telling them what to do. Other agreements might cover what happens at meetings (see pages 135 to 137): how will members take turns to run meetings, give everyone a chance to speak, support careful listening and not interrupt each other, and commit to starting meetings on time. The group may also want to emphasize specific values, such as honest communication, humility, kindness, respect, or sobriety. The group can discuss whether additional people can join and if so, how that should happen.

If the group has been organized through a school or other institution or by an individual with legal requirements to report certain kinds of information to police or government authorities, it is important that everyone understands this before the group starts. Types of situations that may require reporting include a young person talking about harming themselves or saying they have been abused.

Running support group meetings

Sometimes one or two people will be the group leaders and facilitators, but many groups share and rotate these responsibilities among all members.

Beginning the meeting

Beginning each meeting in the same way can help people transition from their previous activities to join in common purpose. Try different ways to start the meeting so the group can decide which they like best. Some groups start with each person saying something they are grateful for. Others start by stretching together, saying a prayer, or taking a few quiet moments to write or draw as a way to gather thoughts and "reset," perhaps in response to the question: "How do you feel right now?" If people check in to say how they are feeling, it may become clear that someone needs special attention that day.

When a group is beginning, it is important to review and remind everyone of the ground rules and see if there are agreements to add or change. When there are new participants, everyone will feel more comfortable when you take time for introductions and give a basic description of how the meeting will proceed.

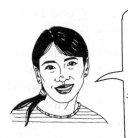

When people don't know each other, invite everyone to mention aspects of their identity they want others to be aware of. For instance, in some groups the introductions include everyone sharing the gender pronoun they use: they, she, or he.

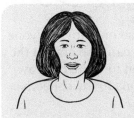

Especially when groups are new, find simple ways to make people feel more comfortable and learn each other's names. For example, ask the group to get up and sort themselves into alphabetical order by first name or by the month they were born. It takes only a few minutes and gets people to talk and accomplish something together.

Encourage participation

Group discussions work best when everyone participates fully and equally, even if this doesn't come naturally to everyone. Good facilitators draw people out and make everyone feel that their ideas are valuable and worth sharing. This is especially important when people have been made to feel shame about aspects of their educational, cultural, or economic backgrounds.

Here are some strategies to encourage participation:

Pay attention to seating. Arrange people to sit in a circle or some other way where everyone can see each other.

Use a talking stick to take turns. An American Indian tradition is to use an object like a talking stick that is passed among speakers. Everyone listens to and does not interrupt the person holding the stick. If the stick comes to a person who does not want to speak, they pass it to the next person.

Give people a moment to prepare their thoughts. Allow time to think quietly before starting a discussion on a major issue or decision. This helps people prepare and feel more confident to speak.

Be aware of people who are quiet or shy. It can take time for people to feel comfortable sharing, so while you should not pressure or force people to participate, you can make it easier. One way is to ask everyone to write questions or comments anonymously and then read them out loud without saying who wrote what. Also, try going around the room giving everyone a turn to speak. Invite shy people by name to speak if you sense they are ready.

Create small groups. Discuss issues in groups of two or three people, then have them report back to the larger group. People may feel more comfortable speaking with only one other person or reporting on a group opinion rather than stating their own.

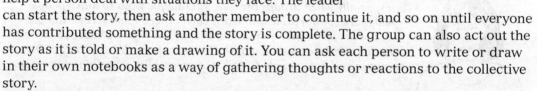

Create a story or drawing. Make up a story about a situation similar to those experienced by members of the group. Hearing about the experiences of others can help a person deal with situations they face. The leader can start the story, then ask another member to continue it, and so on until everyone has contributed something and the story is complete. The group can also act out the story as it is told or make a drawing of it. You can ask each person to write or draw in their own notebooks as a way of gathering thoughts or reactions to the collective story.

Use art, theater, movement, and music. Spark people's creative energy to encourage participation. Drawings, songs, and skits can encourage collaboration among group members and can also be a way for a group to share their ideas with the broader community.

Build capacity and leadership. Allowing people to explore different roles in meetings can help them discover what they are good at. People can take turns leading the group, sending meeting reminders, planning activities, preparing food, or gathering supplies. Sharing different tasks helps people gain experience and encourages involvement from shy people. Draw upon people's strengths and acknowledge everyone's hard work along the way, not just the outcome.

Be a good listener and show interest in what people say (see pages 26 to 27). It may help both individuals and the group if you briefly echo the main point of what a person said so they know they have been understood. Then invite the next person to speak.

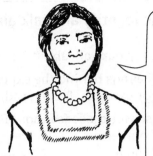

When someone says something that doesn't make sense to me, instead of correcting them or giving my opinion, I ask: "Can you say more about why you believe that?" or "Can you explain more about those feelings?" This shows I value what they have to say and also helps me understand.

A balance of voices. Using terms like "step up" to encourage people who usually speak less, and "step back" for those who tend to talk more, can help build awareness of participation styles. Find kind and direct ways to ask people to step up and step back such as: "Thanks for adding that. Would someone we haven't heard from like to go next?" The group can also talk about how people who know they talk a lot can count to 10 before asking to speak, creating some space for shyer people.

Keep the conversation on topic. If someone strays from the topic, first acknowledge their input: "That's a good point." Then invite them to relate what they were saying to the topic at hand: "How does does that affect you feeling anxious at work?"

Know yourself. Chapter 9, "Helping ourselves to do this work" (see page 143), expands more on how group facilitators and others in a helping role can think through everything they bring to their work. For example, when starting a group or running a meeting, it helps to be aware of your own thoughts and feelings about the topic. Ask yourself: "What about this topic makes me uncomfortable or upset? Do my feelings or experiences affect how well I can listen without judging others? How can I make sure I encourage others to think for themselves without imposing my own opinions?" Also, be aware of how others in the group may see you. Perhaps some women will have a hard time trusting men, or it will feel uncomfortable to have people with one racial, ethnic, or cultural background being directed by someone of another background.

Welcome emotions. Gently encourage people to openly express what they are feeling, recognizing that not all members of the group may feel comfortable opening up until the group has built more trust.

HOW TO   Help people identify and talk about their feelings

Ask questions to help the group talk about feelings and how they affect us:

- What are the main feelings behind the experience just shared with us—what did we hear? For example, feeling sad, helpless, fearful.

- Are there social causes for those feelings? For example, if we were brought up to be ashamed of ourselves or to believe that asking for help shows weakness.

- How is the person coping with these feelings?

- What can we do to provide support?

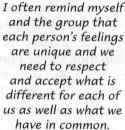

I often remind myself and the group that each person's feelings are unique and we need to respect and accept what is different for each of us as well as what we have in common.

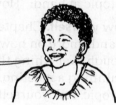

I start meetings by asking everyone to close their eyes, tune into what is happening inside them, and choose 1 to 3 words that express how they're feeling right now.

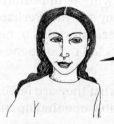

I try to make it easier to talk about emotions by saying: "When I was first told that everything I was feeling meant I had severe depression, I felt even more hopeless." Then I ask: "Did anyone else feel this too? Did anyone feel relief instead?"

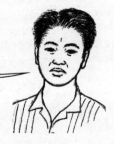

I watch people's body language for clues about what the group needs. If people are looking away, frowning, or dozing off, I ask group members to say how they are feeling or what is going on for them. Then we can all talk about what to do.

When a person in the group shows distress

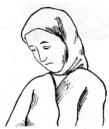

Support group discussions can stir deep feelings. As a person speaks about their thoughts or experiences, they may get very emotional. The group can help the person acknowledge and accept their feelings. The facilitator can say something like: "It's OK, take the time you need, we're here for you." Or they can call on someone else and come back later to the person who was upset.

If a person expresses a more painful or uncontrollable emotion, it may be good to separate the person from the group and talk privately with them to check on their safety, evaluate if there might be a crisis, help them process their emotions, and ask about any other support they may need. You can also ask them if there is something they might want right now that the group can provide. This could be to hear supportive thoughts from others, receive hugs or prayers, decide to sit quietly for a while, or step out of the room to take care of themselves.

If the facilitator leaves the group to pay attention to the person in distress, ask another person to lead the group and check in on how everyone is feeling. The group could discuss the emotions, thoughts, or concerns the group member's distress has brought up for them. Another strategy is to ask everyone to move to a new place in the circle. This literally changes people's point of view and allows a reset.

When the person feels stable enough to participate again or rejoins the group:

- Let the group know what the person said would feel useful to them and limit the group's response or support to that.

- Lead the group in a breathing, moving, or meditative exercise (see pages 31 and 140), or a song or prayer that can unify the group. Be sure to choose an activity that is acceptable to the distressed group member.

- Allow the group to move on naturally, discussing the topic at hand or moving on to another. If this member has a pattern of taking a lot of time and attention, it's OK to openly invite the group to continue: "While David takes his time with this, let's start again with others who are waiting to speak."

- If the group becomes frustrated with the distressed member, it's OK to lead a discussion about those feelings and dynamics. Instead of accusing or blaming them for doing something "wrong," look for a way to have them reflect on what happened, such as: "Can you say more about how you expected us to react when you said that?" This way of "calling in" the person instead of just criticizing them can demonstrate care and an effort to repair the relationships while also building healthy expectations and boundaries for the group.

ACTIVITY   Pause and reset

This can be done individually or as a group. By stopping to relax for 1 to 5 minutes as a group, people can learn how this technique can be used anytime, on their own or when supporting others.

Sit comfortably, feet flat on the floor, hands resting in your lap. Close your eyes.

Ask yourself, "What am I thinking and feeling now?" Notice your thoughts and emotions, and how different parts of your body feel.

Listen to your breath as it goes in and out. Put a hand on your stomach and feel it rise and fall with each breath. Tell yourself, "It's okay. Whatever it is, I am okay." Continue to pay attention to your breath for a while and feel yourself become calmer.

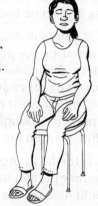

Continue to pay attention to how your body feels and reflect on how you feel overall. Open your eyes and return to the situation, better able to cope.

Not all support groups look the same

Support groups come together for different reasons and what a group does can vary a lot. Groups can create feelings of connection when people feel drawn together by shared identities or have similar life challenges. Support groups do not have to focus on talking, or at least not all the time. Groups can gather to create art or writing or move, dance, or exercise together.

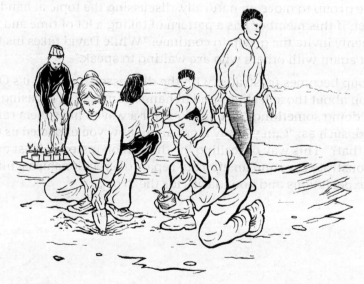

Writing for healing: Telling your story

While no single kind of therapy or group will work for everyone, building trust among group members is critical. That trust often develops more easily among people with shared experiences and shared needs. *The Women's Initiative* of Charlottesville, Virginia, provides a variety of free support groups and counseling using a mix of approaches to meet the unique healing needs of all women, including those who identify as Black, Latina, and LGBTQ+. Their offerings include:

- a group counseling "Sister Circle" program for Black women and other women of color

- a "Life-Giving Gardening" program for people just beginning to plant the seeds of their desired mental health changes

- a Spanish-language *Bienestar* (Well-being) program focusing on self-care skills

- a variety of safe spaces where LGBTQ+ individuals can connect, heal, and have fun

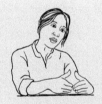

When I saw the notice for this writing group, I thought, "That's not for me! I'm no writer!" But the counselor at The Women's Initiative encouraged me by explaining how the instructor combines meditation and body-based healing practices with an examination of our experiences of adversity and trauma as a way to transform pain into personal growth and healing.

I decided I could at least give it a try. The Writing for Healing facilitator was welcoming, inclusive, encouraging, and not at all pushy. Most of the other women had no experience writing either so I felt no pressure from them, just support. In each session, we would read and discuss a poem or an excerpt from an essay or novel that showed the transforming power of personal storytelling. And we would also try a body-based breathing or stretching exercise to help process the strong emotions we were feeling.

The group made it possible for me to focus my thoughts and put them on paper in a productive and safe way. And it felt good to read my story to the group and then later celebrate the publication of Challenge into Change, a book collecting our writings. That book is a testimony to all who search for the light within to endure hardship on a journey toward hope and healing. Processing painful memories and shaping them into prose and poetry feels bold and empowering. We can share our stories about how we struggle, and share how we find our strength to keep going and to thrive.

9 Helping ourselves to do this work

The work of helping others can be energizing and fulfilling. But sometimes, we can become over-stressed and left feeling overwhelmed or frustrated. Being aware of our own feelings and taking care of ourselves helps us stay healthy and better able to promote social justice, well-being, and mental health for the whole community.

To get through this work, I remind myself of 2 things. First, with the resources I have, I can't help everyone. Second, I will not blame myself for my stress and burnout. Society created this mess and whether I can do a lot or only a little, we are all in this together.

The daily hassles and past hardships of our own lives help define who we are and are part of what makes us good at helping others. They also complicate our interactions with others. The ideas and experiences we bring to a situation include assumptions and prejudices we might not be aware of, so making a space to examine our own issues is important. This is especially true when we are working with others from a different background or culture, and when relations seem more difficult than usual. Noticing how systems and situations create burnout are often first steps to strategies to lower collective stress in our groups and workplaces (see pages 148 to 150).

Noticing how we react to others and what to do about it

People are not as separate from one another as it sometimes seems. We affect one another's emotional and even physical states, often without realizing it. When one person in a room yawns, others may begin to yawn too. Emotional responses, such as impatience, ridicule, being dismissive, and others, also can spread through interactions. Being aware of how your own history and situation may affect or be affected by other people's emotions, frame of mind, and patterns of interacting can help your work with others move forward and avoid getting off track.

Working with people you find "difficult"

If you facilitate groups, are involved in peer counseling, or simply are in contact with lots of people, there will be some you or others find hard to work with. Maybe they ignore what you or others say, talk a lot, or are easily angered. When you find a person "being difficult," try to understand what it is about them that bothers you. Sometimes, it is because our usual way of relating, maybe one we have been trained to do, just doesn't work with them. Sometimes it is because they remind us of someone we had problems with in the past. And sometimes, it is because they limit the participation of others. Whatever the cause, our response to their behavior can make a one-on-one conversation or a group process go off track. It can help to remember:

- The problem is not because of you. The person may be having a bad day, feeling a lot of anxiety, be under extra stress, or have limited social skills. If you are prepared, you can remain calm and tell yourself: "This doesn't have to do with me. They want to draw me in, but I won't let that happen." This can prevent you from responding negatively or with anger to a difficult interaction.

- Even if you don't fully understand why the person is acting a certain way, use your self-awareness to understand why the person is generating a reaction in you, perhaps because of the person's inner "story," (see page 145). Focus on how not to get pulled into an argument or unhelpful exchange.

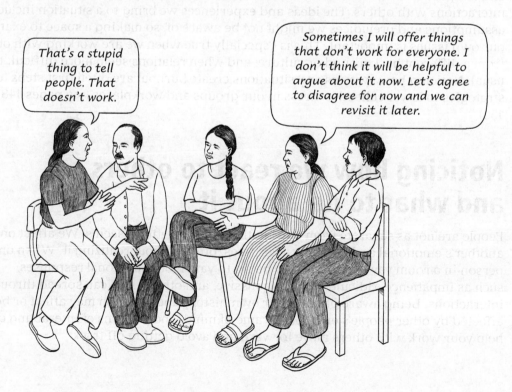

When a person you are trying to help is hard to help. The stress and frustration that often motivates people to look for help can make them interact in less than positive ways. You can aim to set a tone and create an environment that promotes respect, both to and from your co-workers and to and from anyone looking for help. Posting reminders for appropriate respectful behaviors can help—the organization's rules or perhaps a calming or humorous poster on a waiting area wall. But you may also want to have a specific plan about what to do when a person is rude or insults the person trying to help them or others in the space.

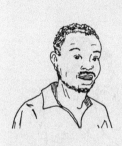

Most staff at our drop-in site for testing street drugs can relate to hardship and try to accept people where they are at. But sometimes people don't love you back. If someone becomes verbally abusive— maybe they say something racist or homophobic—a co-worker will step in immediately and the person who was attacked can leave—it's not their job to put up with it or to defend themselves. The co-worker can say, "We don't talk to people like that and we'd appreciate it if you don't use that language here. That's why she left. I'm going to help you instead. Now what can I do for you?" This is how we signal: "Hey, that's not cool." We want to be clear without further escalating the situation.

HOW TO   Think about people's inner "stories"

A person might not be aware of their behavior patterns or the stories they tell themselves, even when these are a deep part of how they see themselves or what drives them. These patterns can affect what they expect of you or cause you to react a certain way. Here are some examples.

"Everyone betrays me or ends up abandoning me." Sometimes a person is so convinced this always happens to them that they act to make it come true. As a helper, you might think you can change their pattern if you are trustworthy and extra helpful. But if they believe everyone will fail them, they may decide you have let them down no matter what. Instead of telling yourself that you failed, or feeding their belief that you failed, see if instead you can step *outside* their story.

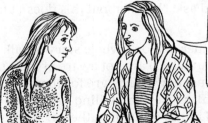

I see that you have lost trust in me. But I will still be here next week and I hope you will be too so together we can keep trying to meet your goals.

HOW TO   Think about people's inner "stories" *(continued)*

"If I'm not the center of attention, I will not get what I need." As good listeners we often try to give people what they want, even those who demand constant attention. But it may never be enough. Meanwhile, others in a group may get frustrated if one person and their needs dominate. This can lead to disruption, provoking the person to leave abruptly to avoid not being the center of attention or cause someone else to leave the group. You may not be able to prevent it, but you may be able to maintain the group by saying something like:

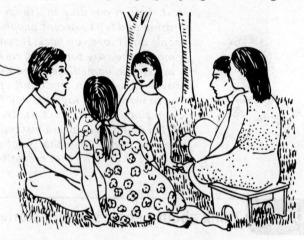

> I am sorry that Anne felt she needed to leave. I'm not sure what happened but it was certainly upsetting. Are people ready to return to what we were discussing or should we first check in on how we are feeling?

> I'm sorry that talking together today has stopped feeling helpful to you. Let's stop for now, but I hope we'll get a chance to try again.

If it is just the two of you when the person gets upset or lashes out, you might just end the interaction for the moment.

There are many other deeply-held stories. If you find yourself acting differently for a person, you may have been pulled into playing a role in their story. Perhaps you are working extra hard for them while paying less attention to the needs of yourself or others. Maybe you find yourself avoiding them, or not giving them your best skills, or showing annoyance. When this begins to happen, take a moment to reflect and ask: "What about this doesn't feel right to me?"

You don't have to figure out the other person's whole story or talk to them about it. Usually, people (including ourselves) are not aware of their powerful inner stories and their effects—it is just how things are for them. It can take a long time for them to change, and unless they are willing to talk openly with you about it, they may feel you are blaming or judging them if you try.

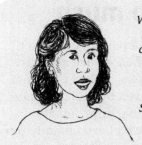

When I see someone has a certain way of being, I figure that's their business. I don't justify my role to them—that's my business! But I can change how I act with them. If I go out of my way a lot to help them, for example, I can change the pattern: "My schedule won't let me continue to make calls to set up your appointments. Maybe someone else can help until you feel OK doing it on your own." Setting limits may lead to the person finding a better solution. But in any case, it helps me stay clear in my role and available to all the people I am committed to helping.

When issues feel too close to our own experiences

Sometimes it can be hard to work with people who are struggling with the same issues we have struggled with ourselves, for example, when a survivor of domestic abuse is supporting someone facing a situation very similar to their experience. Knowing yourself and your reactions, and thinking through your limits can prepare you to better respond.

- Wounds may never completely heal. When yours are touched, how will they trigger your grief or anger? What can you do to prepare for those moments? What support will you need during and after?

- What worked for you might not work for others. Allow each person to find their own path through their situation and toward healing.

- Plan when, how often, and with whom you can talk about how the work makes you feel.

If you find yourself continually reliving your own trauma, you might want to work instead with people whose experiences differ from your own. Or perhaps you can provide support without being the person who listens or counsels directly. It is not a failure to be unhappy doing work that harms you.

Our volunteer peer counseling group helps people who were recently incarcerated and are struggling. Having been there ourselves, we want to help, but some days it can be really hard to listen. We are strict about all counselors meeting every 2 weeks to reflect on our own feelings, to release and process them. Sometimes we talk about setting better boundaries between this work and our own experiences, but mostly we don't focus on "what to do." Just knowing we have this space for ourselves helps.

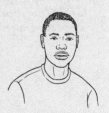

Knowing when the stress is too much

Burnout is a stress overload. It can happen to anyone, whether a parent, caregiver, student, or worker. In many work settings, burnout happens when we are asked to help people with problems caused by conditions—poverty, racism, violence against women, and other structural inequalities—that can only be solved by social change. Even though we may repeatedly improve things for one individual or group at a time, the supply of problems seems never-ending. As if that wasn't hard enough, our organizations and agencies almost always lack the resources we need to do our work well. When our tasks move from being "a challenge" to feeling overwhelming, that's burnout. Although burnout is caused by injustice in the workplace and society in general, it is often experienced as personal failure.

Burnout creates mental and physical exhaustion. For some people, burnout shows in the body with problems such as difficulty sleeping, headaches or other body aches, intestinal problems, or lack of energy. It can create emotional problems like irritability, anger, numbness, an inability to be emotionally involved, and depression. People often feel they must face these difficulties alone and blame themselves for not being good or strong enough, but **the real problem is the conditions causing the burnout**, not you.

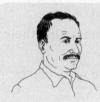

Avoiding burnout means knowing the work we do is hard. We witness people going through overwhelming experiences. To be able to help, we need to be prepared and well-rested. We need to "walk the talk" when it comes to caring for our own wellness and follow the same advice we would give others.

At my office, we have a code word for when our workload, personal life, or their combination becomes too much. "I'm in the ditch" means feeling like you're a truck stuck in the mud. Digging out by yourself is too hard, so let someone throw you a tow rope! When one of us says: "Ditch!" others pitch in right away with help, give you space, or at least make sure you eat lunch! Our supervisors do this too, modeling that it's OK to admit things are "too much" and that looking out for each other is part of our jobs.

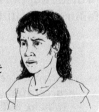

Helping the helpers. When helping people get through health or other problems caused or made worse by inequality and injustice, how is it possible to sustain commitment over a long time? The *Migrant Clinicians Network* (MCN) supports a vast network of health professionals who advocate for and provide services to migrants and others in difficult situations. Within MCN, the Witness to Witness (W2W) Program offers concrete support to health care workers whose care for stressed-out people is itself stressful. The program recognizes the high emotional cost from feeling empathy and compassion day after day, alongside the distress from constantly witnessing the huge harms from systemic and structural causes that don't go away, leading to an endless flow of people who need help.

Witness to Witness sets up peer support groups, offers one-on-one sessions that provide a "listening ear" for clinicians, and helps organizations look at the workplace to see what could make it less stressful.

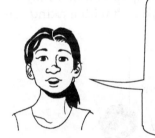

In our work, we talk about "moral injury" to describe what health workers and others go through when their jobs force them to go against their own beliefs. For example, when they can't help a child who needs an expensive medicine and it isn't available to them. The way a lot of people talk about burnout tends to focus on each individual's response to work conditions, whereas "moral injury" directs attention to the conditions themselves.

Though people must depend on their inner resources to get through a bad moment, never forget that "on-the-job stress" is caused by...the job! Solutions come from fixing the workplace and getting the resources that would allow us do our jobs with less stress.

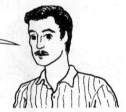

Follow our own advice

"Take care of yourself so you can take care of others." It's so easy to say, but so hard to do! For many of us, it can feel like one more task we don't have time for, one more demand we can't meet.

Just as we look to already-existing strengths, knowledge, and connections to promote community mental health, we can draw on these same resources to address our own stress.

HOW TO   Identify and look for solutions to stress overload

When you know you are not the only one at work or among your friends feeling overwhelmed, you can support each other by talking about what causes your stresses and how to better cope with them, both individually and as a group (see the activity on page 151). Besides describing what causes stress, also focus on what helps relieve it.

- Things you do that help you feel better: walking, playing or watching sports, cooking, reading or writing, engaging with music and art, spiritual practices, gardening, caring for pets. Can you do more of these or do them with others? (See pages 22 to 24.)

- Supportive family, friendships, networks, and community connections: look to your religious or spiritual community, take classes to learn new skills, join groups for recreation, outings, or activism.

- Are there ways you handle stress that you'd like to stop or change? Maybe you and a friend can check in on how each of you is doing with making some changes.

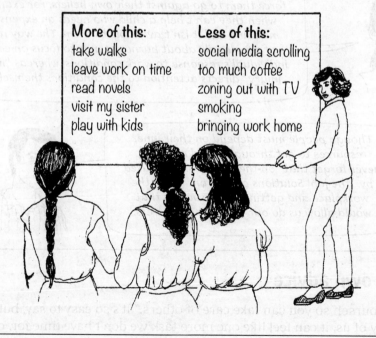

More of this:
take walks
leave work on time
read novels
visit my sister
play with kids

Less of this:
social media scrolling
too much coffee
zoning out with TV
smoking
bringing work home

ACTIVITY   Find stress-busters

Identifying and discussing what we have available to us—our personal strengths, social connections, and other resources—can help to lower the stress in a workplace and for the individuals in it.

1. Discuss these or similar questions as a group:

   - What are your common causes of stress at work?

   - What are the causes of stress for the people you help through your work?

   - How does your stress affect how you work with both your co-workers and the people you help?

   - What do you do to support others in reducing stress?

   - What do you do to help yourself avoid burnout?

2. Have each person fold a piece of paper in 4. Label and list for each section:

   - your **stresses**

   - your **strengths**

   - your **supports**

   - your **stress-busters**

Stresses: work too much long commute	Strengths: humor, tenacious, kind
Supports: church choir, book group, family walks	Stress-busters: baking, dancing, garden, swimming

3. Ask each person to share a few of their examples with the group, then discuss:

   - What do you do in common? What do you do differently? What new ideas will you add to your own list?

   - How can you support each other individually and as a group to reduce stress?

Make time to check in every week or two about what practices lessen the stress, make it worse, or show the need for bigger changes in the workplace.

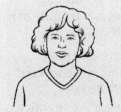

I get fed up with being told to buy scented candles and take a bath. Self-care for me is spending time with friends to do something meaningful and creative, something that reminds me of the strength of working together and being part of a community.

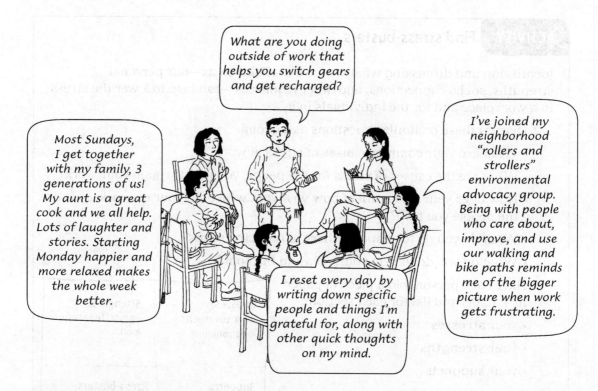

Stronger now, stronger in the long run

Many community-based organizations were created to challenge the inequality and injustice harming people. Many of us working in these groups have a strong moral and political commitment to change unfair conditions and organize people to find solutions.

While there is no shortage of problems that need urgent attention, there is often a great shortage of resources with which to do it. This puts an enormous stress on those of us who earn our living this way. Not only are the salaries and benefits less than in the for-profit world, but the lack of reliable funding makes our jobs unstable. We put up with being understaffed and overworked because we don't want to abandon the people we serve. The injustices are huge and progress is painfully slow. Sometimes it feels like the challenges require superheroes—which we are not.

Supporting community mental health means building organizations and workplaces that encourage participation, don't burn people out, and move toward the social change our communities need, deserve, and demand. While every organization must do this based on their specific situation, these positive practices can improve almost all non-profits and service-oriented organizations:

Support autonomy and reduce hierarchy. Not every organization is suited to a collective structure, and not every person in a workplace wants an equal amount of responsibility. However, workers who control more of the decision-making about their work tend to find ways of working that increase their productivity while decreasing their stress. Give yourself and others the space to adjust work tasks so there is still accountability for doing them, but so they are done in a way that feels more efficient or more rewarding.

More equality in rewards. Large differences in salaries and benefits tell workers that some people are valued more than others. While still rewarding people for seniority, responsibilities, professional credentials, and achievements, a fairer workplace limits salary differences so the gaps are not large. It also creates paths to promotion and changing positions within the organization.

Our organization made a rule that the highest paid person, our Executive Director, cannot be paid more than 2.5 times what the lowest paid, entry-level position earns.

Regional equality. Set salaries to be roughly equivalent to those of other area workplaces. This helps limit turnover and build community.

Paid time off. Especially when jobs are emotionally draining and people struggle to meet client and community needs, time off is a necessity, not a luxury. Besides weekends, make sure there is at least one holiday or other paid day off every month and adequate vacation time. Rest and relaxation keep people able to work for the community, and they don't take anything away from the community. The ability to take personal time for doctor appointments and to care for children or others also keeps anxiety lower.

Look for shared problems that can be solved

Many social change, care-giving, or social service organizations find that it builds morale and improves workplace relations if they can regularly identify and fix workplace issues affecting many people. Involving people from across the organization often generates good, practical ideas about how to make the workplace better. Creating an open culture of addressing problems together can lead to effective and realistic solutions.

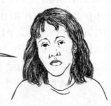

Our intake forms required too much clicking, too many needless questions. They took too much time and worsened ergonomic problems. We cut the form's length in half and changed to software that was much simpler. It was a big relief in our daily work.

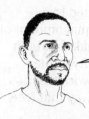

We reactivated a workplace improvement committee. They use anonymous surveys to get feedback, report to our all-staff meetings monthly, and give updates on what is in-progress and what has already been done. It makes us feel more in control of our workplace.

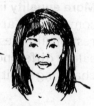

The core of our work is home-based outreach, but policies hadn't been updated in 5 years. Travel costs had risen and we spend more time now with each family. We organized an agency-wide review so policies now match our actual workload and costs.

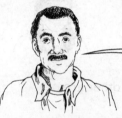

Our unused outdoor patio now has a mural, tables, and a container garden. Many of us now take lunch breaks together. The chance to laugh and know each other better lifts everyone's mood.

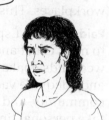

We help people whose lives are really intense. Hearing it day after day can be too much. We get numb to it—our empathy drains away. We now divide the work into administrative work days and days we provide counseling. The result is fewer people quitting due to burnout.

Celebrate ourselves and our victories

So much of our work addresses long-term problems and the need for structural change that we often fail to recognize our small victories, completed projects, and successful transitions out of particularly stressful times. Celebrating with a group lunch, an afternoon off, a trip to a special event, or another enjoyable activity helps build staff unity and the feeling that we are valued for what we do.

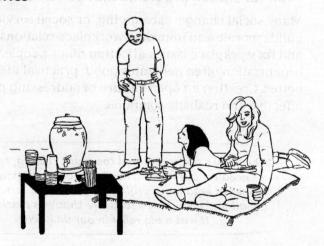

Hotlines, warmlines, and other support

These numbers will connect you to crisis and support services. Add other national, state, or local hotlines or other important emergency phone numbers to the bottom of this list. Share copies with co-workers and neighbors.

988 Suicide and Crisis Lifeline/National Suicide Prevention—call or text 988

Trans Lifeline—call or text 1-877-565-8860

Veterans Crisis Line—dial 988 then press 1 or text to 838255

National Sexual Assault Hotline—1-800-656-HOPE (800-656-4673)

National Domestic Violence Hotline—1-800-799-7233

SAMHSA's National Helpline—1-800-662-HELP (4357)

Gamblers Anonymous—gamblersanonymous.org/u-s-hotlines/ for a list of hotlines by US state

The Trevor Project (to support LGBTQ+ youth)—call 1-866-488-7386, text "START" to 678-678, or chat from: thetrevorproject.org/get-help

Friendly Voice line, call 1-888-281-0145 to leave your information and get a call back. The call back will be from this same number and the caller ID will show "800 Service."

Other important numbers:

_____

_____

_____

_____

_____

_____

Organizations mentioned in this book

AARP Fraud Watch Network, page 126
aarp.org/money/scams-fraud/helpline

AIDS Memorial Quilt, page 44
www.aidsmemorial.org/quilt

Alcoholics Anonymous, page 93
aa.org

Adult Children of Alcoholics (ACA),
page 92
adultchildren.org

Al-Anon, page 92
al-anon.org

Area Agencies on Aging, page 125
eldercare.acl.gov

The Black Doula Project, page 102
blackdoulaproject.com

Black Youth Healing Arts Center,
page 120
irgrace.org/byhac

**Canine Support Teams Prison Pup
Program**, page 56
caninesupportteams.org/prison-pup-
program

Caring Across Generations, page 127
caringacross.org

CHAMACOS, page 99
cerch.berkeley.edu/research-programs/
chamacos-studies

Changing Woman Initiative, page 102
cwi-health.org

Coaching Boys Into Men, page 76
coachescorner.org

Color Splash Out, page 46
colorsplashout.org/about-us

Death Cafe, page 127
deathcafe.com

Debt Collective, page 81
debtcollective.org

Detroit Greenways Coalition, page 12
detroitgreenways.org

Domestic Workers United, page 8
domesticworkersunitednyc.org

**Domestic Abuse Intervention
Programs**, page 73
theduluthmodel.org

**Emerge Counseling and Education to
Stop Domestic Violence**, page 75
emergedv.com

**Faith in Action East Bay, Ceasefire
Initiative**, page 68
fiaeastbay.org/issues/live-free-ceasefire

Family Wellness Warriors, page 78
southcentralfoundation.com/family-
wellness-warriors-nuiju

Flint Public Health Youth Academy,
page 121
cestudioflint.org/youthacademy

Fridays for Future, page 120
fridaysforfutureusa.org

Friendship Line/Friendly Voice,
page 126
ioaging.org/friendship-line-california

Gamblers Anonymous, page 89
gamblersanonymous.org

**Genders & Sexualities Alliance
Networks**, page 46
gsanetwork.org (formerly Gay-Straight
Alliance Network)

The Greening of Detroit, page 12
greeningofdetroit.com

Hijos del Sol Arts Productions, page 99
hijosdelsol.org

Where to find more information

In writing this book, we reviewed many wonderful community-based resources, training guides, and other helpful websites (some already mentioned in this book). Here is a selection of just a few more toolkits and trainings we found inspirational and useful for adaptation.

This list of resources is also available on Hesperian's website. You can view the list by pointing a mobile phone camera at the QR code to the right, or by using this link:

en.hesperian.org/hhg/Other_Resources:Mental_Health

Hesperian's online resources

Hesperian's HealthWiki has free information in many languages (see: en.hesperian.org/hhg/HealthWiki). After opening each page, click "In this chapter" to see related pages.

Where Woman Have No Doctor

Mental health chapter addresses self-esteem, stress, trauma, and community.

• bit.ly/where-women-have-no-doctor-MH

Workers' Guide to Health and Safety

Ideas to promote workplace mental health and advocate for safe and fair workplaces.

• bit.ly/workers-guide-stress-and-MH

Helping Children Live with HIV

Support for children when a caregiver dies, if a child is dying, and for a grieving family.

• bit.ly/helping-children-with-HIV-grief

General mental health

Substance Abuse and Mental Health Services (SAMSHA)

Training tools to prepare for talking about difficult topics with someone needing help (see page 93).

• samhsa.gov/mental-health

U.S. Health and Human Services directory of treatment programs

A resource for persons seeking treatment for mental health concerns and substance use in the US.

- findtreatment.gov

National Alliance on Mental Illness (NAMI)

A starting point for learning about mental illness, includes descriptions of common mental health conditions and many related resources.

- nami.org/nami.org/your-journey

Mental Health America

Mental Health 101 offers information on different conditions, living with mental health concerns, and how to provide support.

- screening.mhanational.org/mental-health-101

Mental Health America BIPOC mental health toolkit

Recognizes the challenges faced by Black, Indigenous, and people of color communities, this toolkit has conversation guides and myth-busting and workshop ideas.

- mhanational.org/bipoc-mental-health/bipoc-mental-health-month/

The Human Rights Campaign

Resource list for LGBTQ+ people of color with emergency resources, treatment options, and specific organizations that can help.

- hrc.org/resources/qtbipoc-mental-health-and-well-being

Peer support

Peer support groups by and for people with lived experience

A booklet distributed by the World Health Organization for planning and starting peer support groups.

- bit.ly/WHOresource-list

A Handbook for Individuals Working in Peer Roles

This downloadable handbook from the Wildflower Alliance gives in-depth advice for peer counseling programs and on how to train and support peer counselors.

- wildfloweralliance.org/books-and-handbooks

National Practice Guidelines for Peer Specialists and Supervisors

By the National Association of Peer Supporters, explains core values of peer helpers and how supervisors can support them.

- bit.ly/practice-guidelines-peer

The Copeland Center

This grassroots movement hub supports community efforts for wellness and recovery by those who have had mental health challenges. It also shares resources for peer support and those becoming certified peer counselors.

• copelandcenter.com/doors-wellbeing/peer-support-resources

Mental health self-help tools

CAPACITAR Emergency Response

Techniques and simple movement and meditation strategies to address trauma and healing.

• bit.ly/Capacitar-emergency-response

How Right Now campaign

Resources to promote and strengthen the emotional well-being and resilience of people facing mental health challenges, including tools for exploring emotions.

• cdc.gov/howrightnow

Helpguide.org

Insightful articles about mental health and guided meditations to reduce stress, increase calm and focus, and promote physical and emotional well-being.

• helpguide.org/mental-health

Skill-building for community work

Community Health Workers (CHWs) Textbook & Training Guide

San Francisco City College's resources to train and support CHWs on mental health and their broader role of supporting community mental health. The textbook is for sale while training guide chapters may be downloaded free.

• bit.ly/foundations-for-CHWS

Witness to Witness (Migrant Clinicians Network)

Resources for people in high-stress jobs working with clients also experiencing high levels of stress, such as asylum seekers, detainees, migrants, and climate refugees.

• migrantclinician.org/witness-to-witness

Healing Justice Trainers' Guide

For healers and organizers to facilitate their own healing justice training as they work to transform systems of state violence.

• justiceteams.org/healing-justice

Children and youth

Say and Play: A tool for young children and those who care about them

From Project Concern International, these activities help children express themselves naturally and help adults understand children.

• bit.ly/say-and-play

The Kaboom! Playbook

Ideas, design guides, and case studies to inspire leaders and change agents creating kid-friendly, playful cities, with equitable access for children of color (see page 108).

• kaboom.org/playbook

People's Movement Center Warriors of Light Kids Yoga in Color

This playlist is a set of videos, 1 to 4 minutes in length, showing age-appropriate yoga techniques for self-calming and empowerment through fun exercise, meditation, and relaxation. Many focus on a specific emotion.

• bit.ly/kids-yoga-in-color

Activities for middle school students

Adapt these art project and other ideas to help young people reflect on their sources of anger and emotions they may find challenging.

• teachingexpertise.com/classroom-ideas/anger-management-activities-for-middle-school

Early Adolescent Skills for Emotions (EASE)

A World Health Organization guide for adolescents and their caregivers, suggests group work to gain skills to reduce distress.

• bit.ly/WHO-EASE-for-youth

Parenting

Mental Health Resources for Parents

Mental Health America's short articles and tips for caregivers including how to talk to kids about many issues, bullying and school settings, parenting with a mental health condition or when also caring for aging parents and others.

• mhanational.org/mental-health-resources-parents

Support for parents of a child with mental illness

This article from Exceptional Lives shows how to be a great friend to parents whose kids are struggling.

• bit.ly/parent-support-resources

American Society for the Positive Care of Children (SPCC)

Offers educational resources, practical tools, and parent coaching to create communities where every child can thrive.

• americanspcc.org/learning-center

Aging

AARP Healthy Aging

AARP guidance on mental health issues that affect older people, including insomnia, loneliness, depression, and how to build community and connections.

• bit.ly/AARP-MH-resource-center

Eldercare Locator

The Administration for Community Living connects people to services for older adults. The "Caregiver Corner" offers information and resources for caregivers.

• eldercare.acl.gov

Addiction

Harm Reduction Resource Center

Offers up-to-date information about evidence-based harm reduction strategies and practices, information on safer drug use.

• harmreduction.org/resource-center

SMART Recovery

This evidence-based recovery method supports people with substance dependencies or problem behaviors to overcome.

• smartrecovery.org

Alcoholics Anonymous (A.A.)

A.A. meetings are free and open to everyone who may struggle with alcohol. The website shows where to find support meetings.

• aa.org

Adult Children of Alcoholics (ACA)

A safe, nonjudgmental environment to share experiences of growing up with abuse, neglect, and trauma, to support healing.

• adultchildren.org

Al-Anon

A mutual support program for people affected by someone else's drinking. Families and friends of alcoholics can make positive changes, whether or not that person admits to a drinking problem or wants help.

• al-anon.org

Substance Use and Misuse in Rural Areas

Examples and guidance for setting up substance use disorder prevention and treatment programs.

• ruralhealthinfo.org/topics/substance-use

Trauma and crisis

A Suicide Prevention Toolkit

Explains what a safety plan is, how they work, how to support a person who wants one, and why they help prevent suicidal behaviors.

• bit.ly/suicide-safety-plan-toolkit

Navigating a Mental Health Crisis

This booklet from the National Alliance on Mental Illness (NAMI) outlines what can contribute to a crisis, warning signs a crisis is emerging, strategies for de-escalation, and suggests resources. Also includes information about advocating for a person in crisis and a sample crisis plan.

• nami.org/support-education/publications-reports

The National Child Traumatic Stress Network (NCTSN)

Describes childhood trauma and information on treatment, practices, and other resources useful for families, health care providers, and advocates.

• nctsn.org/what-is-child-trauma

Violence

Coaching Boys Into Men

Curriculum for schools and sports teams (see page 76), this violence prevention program has activities built around brief weekly team discussions led by the coach.

• coachescorner.org/tools

Interrupting Intimate Partner Violence: A Guide for Community Responses Without Police

Walks organizers through visualizing and planning the formation of a first response team—community members trained to respond to intimate partner violence.

• justiceteams.org/intimate-partner-violence

Domestic Abuse Intervention Programs' "wheel" discussion tool

Developed by battered women discussing the abusive tactics they faced, the Wheel encourages discussion of dangerous forms of power and control in relationships (page 73). This Wheel Gallery shares a variety of wheels that reflect different experiences.

• theduluthmodel.org/wheel-gallery

Pieces of a Bigger Picture: Training Model to Support Victims of Sexual and Domestic Violence

Includes 10 interactive training exercises to help faith leaders (or any reader) better understand trauma, power and control, victim-centered responses, and how to improve support to victims and provide referrals.

• interfaithpartners.org/pieces-of-a-bigger-picture-training

Guidelines Responding to People Who Abuse Intimate Partners

Written for faith leaders, this is useful to anyone encountering people who are the abusers in their relationships. Explores common myths about abusers and suggests what to do when talking with them and other actions to take.

• bit.ly/faith-leader-guidelines

Rape, Abuse & Incest National Network (RAINN)

RAINN (see page 71) provides resources for the person facing sexual violence and for those helping them: what to say and do as well as how to work toward prevention.

• rainn.org

Setting up community programs

Tamarack Institute's Deepening Community network

Upholds community power as a driver of social change. Explains the community assessment process and offers inspiring stories and paths to deepening community.

• bit.ly/Tamarack-building-community

Mental Health Information Community Partnerships Toolkit

This National Institutes of Health resource offers support for communities to address mental health information needs, including practical ways to establish partnerships, develop programs, and promote mental health awareness.

• nnlm.gov/guides/mental-health-information-community-partnerships-toolkit

Rural Mental Health

Developing, implementing, evaluating, and sustaining rural mental health programs.

• ruralhealthinfo.org/toolkits/mental-health

Advocate for Improved Adolescent Health and Well-being

From Women Deliver, a youth-led and youth-serving resource for advocacy, with road maps for policy change.

• bit.ly/adolescent-advocacy-toolkit

Other topics

Rooted in Rights

Stories about disability by disabled people in videos, blogs, and social media campaigns to share perspectives often missing from the conversation.

• rootedinrights.org/stories/blog/topics/mental-health

Movement Generation's Propagate, Pollinate, Practice Curriculum

Toolkit with activities to promote environmental activism and strengthen groups (see page 120).

• movementgeneration.org/propagate-pollinate-practice-curriculum-toolkit

The Farm State of Mind campaign

Addresses anxiety, depression, suicide, and opioid use in the farming community. Combats stigma and provides resources for farmer and rancher mental health.

• fb.org/initiative/farm-state-of-mind

Death Cafe Guide

How-to instructions to organize, advertise, and lead an honest and welcoming group conversation about death (see page 127).

• deathcafe.com/how

A Grassroots Strategy to Transform Long-term Care using Eldercare Dialogues

A report on a series of conversations and a toolkit to walk communities through ways to improve long-term care for their elders (see page 127).

• takerootjustice.org/resources/the-eldercare-dialogues-a-grassroots-strategy-to-transform-long-term-care

Index

NOTE: Find the organizations mentioned in this book on pages 155 to 158, with their page numbers and contact information. All "Activities" and "How to's" are listed at the end of the Table of Contents.

A

Friends and friendships
during adulthood, 122–124
depression and, 45, 47
How to: Pick a health habit, 23–24
mental health helpers and, 150, 151
partner forbidding contact, as abuse, 73
youth activism supported among, 113
also see **Friends support for person with mental health challenges**

Friends support for person with mental health challenges
asking for explanation of unusual behavior, 59
contacting during crisis, 55, 57
monitoring effects of medicines, 50, 51
support given to the friend, 119

G

Gaming addiction, 89
Gang violence, 14, 81
Gender-based violence, 70–78
female genital cutting (FGM/C), 38
sexual orientation and gender identity, 70, 121
also see **Intimate partner violence; Sexual violence**
Gender identity
challenges faced by youth, 46, 112
resources and hotlines, 61, 121
violence based on, 70
also see **LGBTQ+ people**
Generational issues *see* **Intergenerational health issues**
Grief and grieving, 40–44
depression distinguished from, 44–45
How to: Use finger-holding, 21
mass shootings, community grieving, 69
also see **Grief and grieving, blocked**
Grief and grieving, blocked, 42
alcohol/drug use to avoid grief, 42, 90
cultural loss and unresolved grief, 15
Guilt feelings
in depression, 45
in trauma, 34
also see **Blame; Shame**

Gun violence, 68–69
Activity: Speak the unspeakable, 36–37
mass shootings, 34, 69
prevention of, 14, 68, 69
school shootings, 113
young people as aware of, 113

H

Hallucinations, psychosis and, 56, 57, 61, 63, 105
Harm reduction strategies, 95–96
Hate, in news and social media, 69, 113
Headaches, as sign
anxiety, 30
burnout, 148
serious mental illness, 53
stress, 20
trauma, 34
Health care, lack of access, 47, 49–50, 100
also see **Medical care**
Health habits, 23–24
Health insurance
drug/alcohol treatment costs, 93
lack of coverage for mental health, 49
also see **Medicaid; Medicare**
Heart attack vs. panic attack signs, 32
Heart disease, 20
Helping ourselves do this work, 143–154
crisis situations, support following, 65
trauma group facilitators, support for, 37
also see **Burnout**
Hepatitis C, 95
High blood pressure, 20, 24, 80
High school students
anxiety of, and junk food, 24
elders, volunteer with, 125
gender and sexuality, 46
How to: Work with young people, 113
online lives, 114, 115–116
spaces and places to connect, 113
violence prevention and relationships, 76
also see **Youth/adolescence**
History of community
healthy habits, revival of, 24
marking or restoring sites, 7, 44
oral histories, 126

About Hesperian Health Guides

For more than 50 years, Hesperian has provided information and educational tools to equip individuals and community organizations to take greater control over their health and lives and mobilize to eliminate the underlying causes of poor health. Our over 300 resources present easy-to-understand, accurate, culturally respectful, and highly-illustrated information on common health concerns including disease prevention and treatment, environmental health, worker health and safety, child disability, women's health, midwifery, health worker training, and community dentistry. Hesperian publications have been translated and adapted into 85 languages and are used in 221 countries and territories. According to the World Health Organization (WHO), our best-known publication, *Where There Is No Doctor*, is the most widely used health manual in the world.

How this book was developed

The creation of *Promoting Community Mental Health* and all our other resources is the result of a collaborative model that solicits as much input as possible from both grassroots partners and experts. A diverse network of partner organizations and volunteers provided feedback to help us develop, test, and improve this book. You can help us further improve this resource by sending your ideas, feedback, and suggestions to MentalHealth@hesperian.org

Support our work

Hesperian resources are published in English, Spanish, and many other languages; they are available in print and digital formats, including mobile apps, PDFs, and our free online HealthWiki.

As a not-for-profit organization, Hesperian's work is made possible through your book purchases and donations. To support further development and translations of *Promoting Community Mental Health* and other vital health information, please visit hesperian.org/donate for ways to give. See some of our resources on the following pages and visit our website: hesperian.org

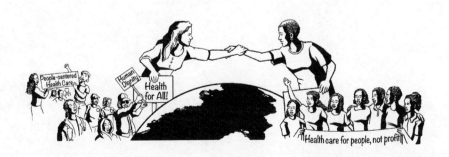

Other Books from Hesperian

Hesperian resources are available in English, Spanish, and a variety of other languages. See the Language Hub on our website (hesperian.org) to find materials in your language.

Health Organizing and Training

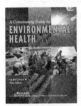

A Community Guide to Environmental Health provides tools, knowledge, and inspiration to help health promoters, activists, and community leaders take charge of their environmental health. This comprehensive guide supports urban and rural communities and covers topics from toilets to toxics, watershed management to waste management, and agriculture to air pollution. Informative case studies, impactful activities, and how-to instructions empower people to address environmental health hazards where they live and work. 617 pages, paperback.

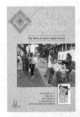

Recruiting the Heart, Training the Brain tells the story of how Latino Health Access developed its groundbreaking promoter model of peer-to-peer outreach and education in Santa Ana, California. Facing problems such as obesity and diabetes, exacerbated by poverty and discrimination, their strategies, advice, and accomplishments inspire hope and change across an increasingly unhealthy country. 280 pages, paperback.

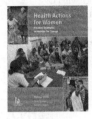

Health Actions for Women addresses social factors that prevent women and girls from enjoying healthy lives. It contains a wealth of clearly explained and engagingly illustrated activities, stories, and strategies to help women and men facilitate community discussions and action. User-tested by 41 groups in 23 countries, this resource offers proven strategies to help improve women's social status and health outcomes, even in challenging settings where organizing for women's health is difficult or dangerous. 330 pages, paperback.

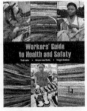

Workers' Guide to Health and Safety makes occupational safety and health accessible to those most affected by physical, social, and economic hazards—the workers themselves. Actionable tools and strategies support workers, supervisors, safety committees, and labor relations courses to improve workplace experiences and overall well-being for workers. The insights and techniques are useful in any factory, and especially in the garment, shoe, and electronics industries. 576 pages, paperback.

Reproductive and Women's Health

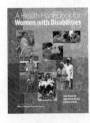

A Health Handbook for Women with Disabilities provides individuals and caregivers suggestions on caring for daily needs, healthy and safe sexual relationships, family planning, pregnancy and childbirth, and defense against violence, abuse, and stigma. This groundbreaking guide helps women with disabilities overcome barriers to poor health and advocate for better care. 384 pages, paperback.

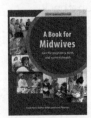

A Book for Midwives covers the essentials of care before, during, and after birth. A vital resource for practitioners, training programs, and anyone interested in safer birthing. Clearly written and illustrated, this book discusses preventing, managing, and treating obstetric complications, covers HIV in pregnancy, birth, and breastfeeding, and has expanded information on reproductive health care. 527 pages, paperback.

188

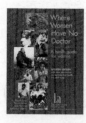

Where Women Have No Doctor combines self-help medical information with an understanding of the ways poverty, discrimination, and cultural beliefs limit women's health and access to care. Clearly written and with over 1000 drawings, this essential resource addresses health issues across the lifespan and considers issues specific to girls, older women, women with disabilities, and refugees. 583 pages, paperback.

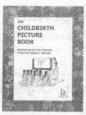

The Childbirth Picture Book provides a simple and complete guide to the basics of conception, pregnancy, childbirth, and breastfeeding. This short resource contains detailed line drawings depicting every step of the reproductive process. 68 pages, staple-bound booklet.

Early Assistance

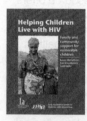

Helping Children Live with HIV is an innovative community health guide designed to ensure children with HIV can grow to adulthood and live full lives. Richly illustrated, the practical advice in this book addresses both the physical and emotional health needs of children living with HIV, and helps parents, caregivers, and health workers provide them with the love and support they deserve. 315 pages, paperback.

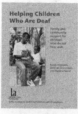

Helping Children Who Are Deaf focuses on care for young children who do not hear well and explores ways that communities can work to support children with hearing difficulties. Chapters include information to aid parents and caregivers to assess hearing loss, explore causes of deafness, and learn basic communication using both signed and spoken methods of communication. 250 pages, paperback.

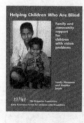

Helping Children Who Are Blind is an important aid for parents and other caregivers helping children with vision problems, starting from birth and through age 5, to develop all their capabilities. Topics include assessing how well a child can see, preventing blindness, moving around safely, teaching common activities, and more. 192 pages, paperback.

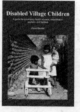

Disabled Village Children is a comprehensive resource covering common disabilities of children. It suggests community-based rehabilitation activities and explains how to make a variety of low-cost aids with local resources in mind. Emphasis is placed on how to help disabled children find a role and be accepted in the community. 654 pages, paperback.

More Books and Booklets

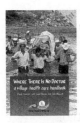

Where There Is No Doctor, perhaps the most widely used health care manual in the world, provides vital, easily understood information on how to diagnose, treat, and prevent common diseases. An emphasis is placed on prevention, including cleanliness, diet, vaccinations, and the important role of the individual and community in health care. 446 pages, paperback.

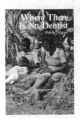

Where There Is No Dentist shows how to care for teeth and gums at home and in community and school settings, including prevention of dental issues through hygiene, nutrition, and education. The book also includes detailed and illustrated information on using dental equipment, placing fillings, taking out teeth, and material on HIV/AIDS and oral health. 248 pages, paperback.

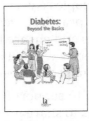

Diabetes: Beyond the Basics is for people living with diabetes, family members, health workers and those working to prevent new cases of diabetes in their communities. Expanded from material in *Where There Is No Doctor*, this booklet addresses both the physical and social issues tied to diabetes and provides thoughtful discussion questions for health educators and self-help groups. 44 pages, staple-bound booklet.

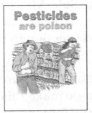

Pesticides are Poison provides detailed information about the health effects of pesticides. In addition to how to read pesticide labels, this short resource addresses how to treat people in pesticide emergencies and reduce harm caused by pesticides. It also offers alternate pest control methods that do not use harmful chemicals. Excerpted from *A Community Guide to Environmental Health*. 38 pages, staple-bound booklet.

See our website: hesperian.org for many more books, booklets, and online resources.

Ordering from Hesperian

We provide bulk ordering discounts to bookstores, schools, non-profits, universities, and other organizations.

To purchase books, visit: store.hesperian.org
email: bookorders@hesperian.org
or call: 510-845-4507.

For more information about review or exam copies, or to apply for our Gratis Books Program which distributes free copies of Hesperian's community health books to health workers, teachers, and local leaders in low-income communities, please email: hesperian@hesperian.org or visit: hesperian.org.

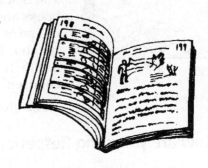

190

Reproductive Health Apps

Each month, thousands of people rely on Hesperian's suite of multilingual reproductive health apps for practical, clear, and trustworthy information to make confident informed decisions and ensure healthier outcomes for themselves and for others. The free apps operate without an internet connection or data plan once installed on a device and do not collect personal information.

Family Planning - Designed to support frontline health workers, community leaders, and health advocates to share unbiased information on birth control options. A built-in "Method Chooser" can help determine which methods best match individual preferences, circumstances, and health history.

Safe Abortion - Written in easy-to-understand and nonjudgmental language, the Safe Abortion app can help people needing or giving abortion and post-abortion care. Now in 11 languages, with a read-aloud function in select languages.

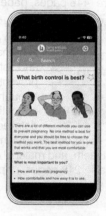

Safe Pregnancy and Birth - Find accurate, easy-to-understand information on pregnancy, birth, and care after birth. Clear illustrations and plain language make this award-winning app practical and user-friendly for community health workers, midwives, and individuals and families.

All apps can also be used without needing to download them. Access them online through a secure web browser at **hesperian.org/mobile-apps**

Free Health Information Online

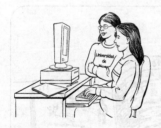

The Hesperian HealthWiki is an online library of Hesperian resources in many languages.

The HealthWiki offers free digital access to Hesperian books and fact sheets. Read essential health information online or, to easily share, print a page or download a chapter. Topics include environmental health, reproductive health, health rights advocacy, and the health of women, children, workers, and people with disabilities.

en.hesperian.org/hhg/HealthWiki

How are you using Hesperian resources?

Please tell us! We would love to hear how our resources enable you to make positive change.

hesperian.org/share-your-story